TRUE OR F

If my cholesterol level is low, I don't have to worry about heart disease.

False. Although your cholesterol level is one important factor in determining risk for heart disease, there are many others. More than half of all heart attacks occur in people with normal cholesterol levels.

If I had other risk factors for   art disease, my doctor would tell me.

Not necessarily. Many   focus on treating   ing illnesses, not on preventing them. If your cholesterol and blood pressure are normal, you don't smoke, and you appear to be otherwise healthy, your doctor may not look any deeper.

Doctors don't believe in alternative treatments for heart disease.

False. Over the past two decades, scientific research has demonstrated the efficacy of alternative therapies, and many doctors now embrace such natural approaches as dietary changes, exercise, vitamins and other supplements, and mind-body relaxation techniques. Some patients can avoid prescription medications entirely and control their risk of heart disease through lifestyle changes and natural treatments.

TAKE CONTROL OF YOUR HEART'S HEALTH WITH...
WHAT YOUR DOCTOR MAY NOT TELL YOU ABOUT™ *CHOLESTEROL*

"A must-read if your cholesterol is high and you are trying to decide what to do about it. Dr Stephen Devries shares his twenty years of clinical experience as an integrative cardiologist and clearly guides patients through the myriad of supplement, herbal, dietary, and medication options for cholesterol management."

—Victoria Maizes, M.D., executive director,
Program in Integrative Medicine, University of Arizona

"It is so refreshing to work with a cardiologist who embraces prevention based on state-of-the-art medical tests and then uses these results to plan a heart-healthy diet and supplement and protocol. I have said many times that we need to clone Dr. Devries. This book will help accomplish that goal."

—Bonnie C. Minsky, M.A., M.P.H., L.D.N., C.N.S.,
wellness director, Nutritional Concepts, Inc., author of
Nutrition in a Nutshell and *Our Children's Health*

"A very practical and science-based approach to utilizing diet and natural products to lower their risk for heart disease...Utilizing his years of experience in integrative medicine, Dr. Devries provides the latest practical information for the person who desires alternative and medically valid prevention therapy."
—Michael H. Davidson M.D. F.A.C.C., professor of medicine,
director of preventive cardiology, Rush University
Medical Center, Chicago, IL

WHAT YOUR DOCTOR MAY *NOT* TELL YOU ABOUT™
CHOLESTEROL

The Latest Natural Treatments and Scientific
Advances in One Breakthrough Program

STEVEN R. DEVRIES, M.D.
with
WINIFRED CONKLING

A Lynn Sonberg Book

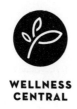

**WELLNESS
CENTRAL**

NEW YORK   BOSTON

PUBLISHER'S NOTE: The information herein is not intended to replace the services of trained health professionals or be a substitute for medical advice. You are advised to consult with your health care professional with regard to matters relating to your health, and in particular regarding matters that may require diagnosis or medical attention.

Copyright © 2007 by Stephen R. Devries, M.D. and Lynn Sonberg
All rights reserved. Except as permitted under the U.S. Copyright Act of 1976, no part of this publication may be reproduced, distributed, or transmitted in any form or by any means, or stored in a database or retrieval system, without the prior written permission of the publisher.

The title of the series What Your Doctor May *Not* Tell You About . . . and the related trade dress are trademarks owned by Grand Central Publishing and may not be used without permission.

Wellness Central
Hachette Book Group
237 Park Avenue
New York, NY 10017

www.HachetteBookGroup.com

Printed in the United States of America

First Edition: June 2007
10 9 8 7 6 5 4 3

Wellness Central is an imprint of Grand Central Publishing.
The Wellness Central name and logo is a trademark of Hachette Book Group, Inc.

Library of Congress Cataloging-in-Publication Data
Devries, Stephen R.
      What your doctor may not tell you about cholesterol : the latest natural treatments and scientific advances in one breakthrough program / Stephen R. Devries, with Winifred Conkling.—1st ed.
      p. cm.
      Includes index.
      ISBN 978-0-446-69773-6
      1. Hypercholesteremia—Prevention—Popular works. 2. Heart—Diseases—Prevention.
3. Cholesterol—Physiological effect. I. Conkling, Winifred. II. Title.
RC632.H83D48 2007
616.3'99705—dc22   2006025862

Book design by Charles Sutherland

For my father,
Robert Devries,
of blessed memory,
who will always be my beloved teacher and inspiration.

For my mother,
Helen Devries,
whose strength and love light my way.

In Gratitude

M ost thanks are due to my wonderful wife, Pam, who gave me boundless love and support to write this book in the midst of our busy family life. To my son Josh, whose radiant spirit and determination to overcome challenges is a role model for me. To my son Andy, whose keen insight and kindness is a joy to behold and always makes me proud.

I owe a great deal of gratitude to my friends and colleagues, who have been my sounding board and encouraged me to follow my dream to a different path in medicine. I would especially like to acknowledge the friendship and support of Ryan Gantes, Julie Esguerra, Mary McGarrigle, and Marianne Riley-Jensen.

My deep appreciation to the teachers of my integrative medicine training—an experience that has enriched my life immeasurably. Special gratitude to Andrew Weil for sharing with me his expansive vision of integrative medicine and for his personal support and invaluable assistance in reviewing the outline of this book. Special thanks to Victoria Maizes for her friendship and outstanding leadership skills in directing the groundbreaking integrative medicine program at the University of Arizona. I would also like to thank Tieraona Low Dog for sharing with me her bottomless fund of botanical knowledge and for her expert review of the chapter on supplements—as well as for her constant enthusiasm and good cheer.

Very special thanks to Lynn Sonberg for connecting me with Warner Wellness to write this book, and for her thoughtful suggestions along the way. Many thanks also to Leila Porteous for her editorial expertise and care in attending to countless details.

My profound gratitude is extended to Winifred Conkling, an exceptionally talented writer and researcher, who worked very closely with me in the preparation of this book.

Contents

Introduction

Are you at risk of a heart attack? You may be, and for reasons that you—and your doctor—may not realize. First, the good news: Heart disease is largely preventable. By some estimates, eight out of ten heart attack deaths can be prevented. All too often, however, doctors miss these opportunities for prevention.

Cholesterol receives a lot of deserved attention as a leading cause of heart disease, but the connection between cholesterol and heart disease is more complicated than many doctors realize. Although cholesterol is one very important factor in determining your heart attack risk, it is by no means the only one. I have seen thousands of heart patients over almost twenty years of practice, and as director of the Integrative Program for Heart Disease Prevention at the University of Illinois, I have seen firsthand that many people suffer heart attacks with what appears to be a perfectly desirable cholesterol level.

To truly understand if you are at risk, you must examine a range of risk factors that go beyond cholesterol. Too often, these additional markers are not checked, resulting in false assurances that all is well and missing the opportunity to prevent heart disease before it becomes worse. Understanding the many markers for heart disease and the expanding world of treatments—including natural options—is critical to keeping your heart healthy.

USING THIS BOOK

What Your Doctor May Not *Tell You About Cholesterol* will give you information about a new integrative approach to heart disease prevention that combines the best of traditional approaches with the most successful natural treatment options that have passed scientific scrutiny. You will learn about a number of powerful treatments that will help you maintain optimal cholesterol levels, as well as optimize other risk factors.

The book is divided into two parts:

- Part 1, "Are You at Risk of a Heart Attack?," provides a thorough explanation of the tests that can be used to assess your heart health, including both traditional cholesterol tests and newer blood markers that can offer essential information about your cardiovascular condition. It includes information on what the tests measure, what the results mean, and how the tests should be administered.
- Part 2, "Take Action," offers practical information on how to take steps to lower your risk of heart attack. Based on the results of the tests explored in part 1, you can customize an approach to heart health that targets your specific areas of concern. The chapters cover the ways that supplements, diet, lifestyle changes, and medications can be used to lower cholesterol and improve other cardiac risk markers.

In addition, to make it easy to review the concepts presented throughout the book, the final entry of each chapter is a section titled "Take This to Heart," which provides a summary of the key facts.

The book can be read cover to cover or used as a reference to explore options on a specific topic. If you are concerned about your overall risk of a heart attack because you have a family history of heart disease, you might prefer to review all five chapters in part 1, so that you will be armed with the information you need to discuss with your doctor the specific blood tests and procedures that can more fully assess your cardiac health.

If, on the other hand, you are curious about the use of coenzyme Q10, you could turn directly to chapter 6, "Supplements for a Healthy Heart," where you will find an overview of what the supplement is and how it can be used to lower cholesterol and prevent heart disease. Those readers who wish to know more about specific research findings will find complete citations to journal articles and other references of interest in "Chapter Notes" at the back of the book.

A FINAL WORD

The information presented in this book is based on my twenty years of experience working with thousands of cardiac patients. Often patients ask me if I take my own good advice: I do. For fifteen years, I have been a vegetarian (although I do eat dairy and fish), I take daily nutritional supplements (a multivitamin, fish oil, vitamin C, and vitamin D), I do not smoke, and I strive to exercise as much as possible. (I confess: Consistent exercise is my toughest health challenge!) I practice relaxation techniques, and I have recently enjoyed the benefits of healing touch and Reiki.

I believe that the information presented in this book can help you minimize your risk of heart attack and improve your overall health. However, it does not replace the need for professional medical care. I encourage you to discuss the suggestions listed here with your doctor and other health care professionals so that you can manage your cholesterol and other cardiac risk factors in a way that embraces the best of both conventional and complementary medicine.

WHAT YOUR DOCTOR
MAY *NOT* TELL YOU
ABOUT™
CHOLESTEROL

PART 1

Are You at Risk of
a Heart Attack?

Chapter 1

What Your Doctor May *Not* Tell You

Five years ago, the well-known coach of a Chicago professional sports team came to see me because he was concerned about his risk of having a heart attack. One look at him and you'd think he was worried about nothing: At age forty-six, he was fit and trim; he didn't smoke; his blood pressure was normal; he had no history of diabetes; and his cholesterol levels appeared very desirable.

Still, the coach did have one significant risk factor: Ten male members of his immediate family had died of heart disease before age fifty-three. This remarkable family history gave him cause for concern, but one doctor after another had looked him over and told him that he was in excellent shape; no problem could be identified. These physicians offered no treatments and recommended no lifestyle changes.

Of course, there were steps the man could take to minimize his risk, but to identify them his doctors needed to look a little deeper into his health profile. When the coach came to my office, I performed a series of blood tests, including several that his previous physicians hadn't recommended. The results: His

Lp(a) level—a genetically determined risk factor for heart disease—was six times the upper limit of normal. It was, at that time, the highest level I had ever seen. Left untreated, this imbalance would have left him at great risk of heart attack. Fortunately, his Lp(a) level has since improved with treatment, hopefully giving him the opportunity to escape the fate of his relatives.

If this coach had relied on conventional cardiovascular tests—remember, his cholesterol profile was desirable—he may never have learned that he was, in fact, at great risk of heart attack. Millions of Americans share the same fate: They are at high risk of heart attack despite having normal cholesterol levels. In fact, *more than half of all heart attacks occur in people with normal cholesterol levels.*

Each year, about 650,000 Americans suffer their first heart attack. Many of these people have been careful about diet and exercise and have never had any cardiac symptoms. About half of them have had a recent medical checkup that indicated that their cholesterol levels were normal. Clearly, to know your risk of heart attack, you must look at more than your basic cholesterol numbers.

BEYOND CHOLESTEROL

Elevated cholesterol is a significant risk that should not be ignored. If a patient comes to me with elevated cholesterol, I recommend he or she take steps to lower it, often by starting with the natural options described in this book. Still, the standard cholesterol tests are incomplete when it comes to determining risk. In order to dig deeper and identify risks hidden by the routine cholesterol profile, additional tests that go beyond cholesterol are needed. (These specific tests are described in detail in chapter 4.)

If cholesterol isn't the all-encompassing risk factor many doctors make it out to be, why don't other physicians look beyond cholesterol to other risk factors? In my opinion, there are two main reasons:

- Many doctors don't emphasize prevention. Instead, the focus tends to be on treatment of existing medical problems. I believe it makes a lot more sense to prevent heart problems than to treat them after the fact.
- Fewer data are available for the newer risk markers of heart disease than for standard cholesterol tests. Yet it's clearly recognized that more than one out of three patients with a heart problem has a normal cholesterol level. Obviously, factors beyond cholesterol play a significant role in bringing on heart disease.

DISCOVERING ALTERNATIVES

In the past decade or so, patients have led their doctors toward a deeper appreciation of alternative therapies, those approaches to healing not traditionally taught in medical schools. According to the National Center for Complementary and Alternative Medicine, a branch of the National Institutes of Health that was founded in 1998, more than one out of every three Americans uses some form of complementary medicine.

Of course, alternative therapies aren't new; many of the "newly discovered" approaches to healing have in fact been used for thousands of years by other cultures. The new wrinkle involves integrative medicine, an approach to patient care that involves a combination of conventional medicine and natural approaches, including simple yet powerful dietary changes, exercise, vitamins, supplements, and mind–body relaxation techniques. In my opinion, integrative medicine makes the most sense and will be the medicine of the future. Why shouldn't both doctors and patients embrace the best of both conventional and alternative therapies?

My belief in integrative medicine has been affirmed by my experiences with the heart disease prevention program at the University of Illinois. When we launched this program, my colleagues and I first focused on reducing cholesterol with medication. Over time, the same patients returned with ongoing symptoms of heart disease despite our best efforts. It became clear that our approach to treatment—however valuable in some circumstances—was woefully incomplete. Although the powerful medications we relied upon did a great job at lowering LDL (the "bad" cholesterol), we were not addressing a host of other (often inherited) risk factors. There was more to the story.

I was able to explore these other risk factors when I opened the Healthy Heart Center, a suburban satellite of the University of Illinois in Deerfield, Illinois, dedicated exclusively to heart disease prevention, one of the first such sites in the nation. Many of my patients in this Deerfield site were very interested in exploring more natural approaches to heart health. They often asked me: "I am willing to use medicine as a last resort, but can't we first try something else before a prescription?"

My interest in seeking natural treatment options led me to embark on a new path, one that eventually led me to additional training in integrative medicine in a two-year program led by Dr. Andrew Weil. This amazing experience was like entering medical school a second time, allowing me to appreciate an expanded approach to wellness and healing.

In my role as a prevention specialist, I try to provide a link between conventional and alternative approaches to heart health, a rare combination, especially in academic centers.

Some patients feel comfortable working with me because I am a conventionally trained cardiologist perfectly willing to use prescription medications and recommend cardiac procedures when necessary. Other patients choose to see me because I am an enthusiastic advocate for the use of natural approaches to disease prevention and management when appropriate. My goal is to provide optimal treatment for all of my patients, and, in turn, to introduce a broader philosophy of healing to patients who may have been using only half the resources available to them.

My patients are also my teachers, often educating me about new natural treatment possibilities. I believe that many alternative treatments can provide important benefits for prevention of heart disease, although I do believe that all methods—both traditional and complementary—need to be carefully reviewed and used under the supervision of a doctor overseeing total patient care.

Unfortunately, too many doctors discourage patients from exploring alternative treatments. One patient who came to see me had been advised by a chiropractor to take nutritional supplements to aid in her mild depression. The treatment worked beautifully; she reported that she "never felt better." Her internist, a man she had trusted with her health concerns for ten years, declared that he would no longer be her physician if she continued to use the supplements. She reported feeling manipulated and insulted by his lack of respect for her health choices, so she left his practice. I wish I could say that this is an isolated incident, but there are too many stories of patients who are treated similarly. The negativity and ridicule that some patients face from their physicians when they discuss natural treatments help explain why a majority of patients who use alternative treatments choose not to tell their physicians about these treatments.

Of course, I strongly recommend that you discuss your entire medical history with your doctor. To prevent side effects or drug interactions, it is especially important that you review any special diet programs or supplements you are considering. If your doctor is concerned about the specific risks of a complementary treatment you are receiving or feels that more traditional therapy is urgently needed, I encourage you to listen carefully to his or her recommended changes. If, on the other hand, your physician ridicules your choices or discounts your treatment without a specific reason, I would consider looking for a more open-minded doctor.

NATURAL TREATMENTS WORK

The majority of patients who come to see me want to avoid prescription drugs when possible. They tend to be goal-oriented people who are willing to make the lifestyle changes necessary to improve their overall health. If you can manage your cardiovascular risk factors naturally, so much the better. I write plenty of prescriptions for statins and other cholesterol medications, but I also recommend that my patients use natural treatments. In my experience, patients who do need medications—and use natural treatments as well—tend to need lower doses and have much better control of their condition than those who use prescription medications alone.

It typically takes several months to note a measurable

change in cholesterol levels using lifestyle and natural treatments. For patients with moderately elevated cholesterol, I monitor them every two to three months to determine whether the problem is responding to lifestyle changes and complementary treatments. Of course, the higher a patient's cholesterol level, the greater my concern about lowering it quickly; in patients with very high cholesterol, I may recommend both lifestyle changes and the use of prescription medications until the problem is brought under control.

This book will help you identify your risk of having a heart attack (part 1) and help you take steps to minimize those risk factors using natural methods (part 2). Part 2 also includes a discussion of the safe and effective use of prescription medications, which may be an essential part of your treatment program.

Before I tell you how to lower your cholesterol levels, it is important for you to understand what cholesterol is and the role it plays in your overall health. Chapter 2 describes the role of inflammation and cardiovascular disease, and provides a summary of the evidence linking cholesterol and heart disease. Chapter 3 explains the various types of cholesterol and its role in the body, followed by a detailed explanation of traditional cholesterol testing.

TAKE THIS TO HEART

- The routine cholesterol profile is an important, but incomplete, measure of cardiac risk.
- In my view, the optimal approach to wellness and healing is integrative medicine, a combination of conventional medicine and natural approaches,

including dietary changes, exercise, vitamins, supplements, and mind–body relaxation techniques.
- Your doctor should be aware of all the treatments
  you receive, from both conventional and alternative providers.

———— ◆•◆ ————

Chapter 2

Inflammation, Cholesterol, and Heart Disease

In my practice, I encounter two types of patients: those who want to understand everything there is to know about heart disease and those who want to be spared the details and simply follow a treatment program. This chapter is for those of you who want to understand the fascinating mechanics of heart disease and how cholesterol and inflammation contribute to cardiovascular problems. If you're the second type of patient—one who wants to skip the physiology and move on to the nuts and bolts of cholesterol testing—then move on to chapter 3, which will describe cholesterol testing and how to understand what your results really mean.

THE TRAFFIC JAM IN YOUR CIRCULATORY SYSTEM

Your body has an amazing challenge: to supply oxygen-enriched blood to nearly every cell, estimated at up to one hundred trillion, every minute of every day. This occurs through a complex network of more than twelve thousand

miles of arteries, veins, and capillaries. Your heart is the pow-
erhouse of this system, meeting the never-ending demand for
oxygen by beating about a hundred thousand times a day and
pumping more than one thousand gallons of blood.

Cardiovascular disease refers to traffic problems in this delicate cardiovascular highway. Narrowing of the arteries from
plaque buildup causes a bottleneck that limits blood flow and
causes a shortage of its precious oxygen cargo. When the slow-
down occurs in lanes leading to your heart, you could develop
chest pain or irregular heartbeats. If the oxygen traffic stalls in
the arteries leading to your brain, you may temporarily lose the
ability to speak or move your legs. In the worst case, a sudden
crack develops in the "pavement" of the artery, causing the
flow of blood to come to a complete stop. A blockage in blood
flow to the heart leads to a heart attack, and a breakdown in
the arteries leading to the brain causes a "brain attack," or
stroke. The technical term for a heart attack—*myocardial
infarction*—comes from the words *myocardium,* meaning
"heart muscle," and *infarct,* which refers to an area of dead
tissue.

The process by which blood vessels narrow, or *atherosclerosis,* is a gradual one typically spanning many decades. Early
stages of this process can appear in children under ten years
old, in whom fatty streaks have been documented in previously pristine arteries. The early stages of this process occur
gradually as the plaque slowly narrows the artery, similar to
the mineral deposits that eventually line household plumbing.
It is a commonly held belief that severe heart disease does not
develop until midlife or later. A surprising study of young ca-
sualties during the Korean and Vietnam wars indicates otherwise: At an average age of twenty-six years, more than
75 percent had some degree of atherosclerosis in their hearts,

with one out of five soldiers having more than a 50 percent narrowing.

Until fairly recently, most experts believed that a heart attack was the result of a purely mechanical problem in which blood congealed at the site of a severe narrowing, completely blocking the flow. This idea, of cholesterol buildup as an inert roadblock, has recently undergone a major revision. Like a volcano that is brewing but has not yet erupted, plaques look disarmingly rigid, but in fact they have a very active—and dangerous—inner life.

INFLAMMATION: FRIENDLY FIRE AIMED AT THE HEART

Only recently have cardiologists begun to appreciate the role of inflammation in triggering the process that makes a seemingly stable plaque erupt into a fatal heart attack. Inflammation is the body's response to injury—the call to arms that allows it to muster an infantry of white blood cells, the same response needed to fight off infection.

The first stage of plaque formation involves injury to the delicate lining of the artery called the intima. To defend against the damage, white blood cells—typically monocytes and T-cells—gather at these injured sites and stick to the cell walls. These monocytes do a Dr. Jekyll and Mr. Hyde transformation to become macrophages, which have a voracious appetite for LDL cholesterol floating by in the bloodstream. When macrophages feast on large helpings of LDL, they become foam cells, which—when gathered together in the lining of the artery—appear as fatty streaks. Fatty streaks are the earliest stages of plaque and can be found in people of all ages.

If the cause of the inflammation—such as high cholesterol,

smoking, or obesity—is not brought under control, the inflammatory response continues, causing the plaque to grow larger. Arteries diseased in this way have an amazing self-preservation strategy: As the plaque grows, the artery stretches open to maintain a normal amount of blood flow. As the plaque builds up, it develops a fibrous cap, similar to a scab over a cut. As long as this coating remains stable, it is not an immediate threat. However, if the fibrous cap ruptures, the plaque is exposed and the body responds by forming a clot that causes a heart attack. The macrophage, a key cell in the inflammatory process, secretes an enzyme that thins and weakens the fibrous cap, increasing the likelihood of rupture. High blood levels of two substances—C-reactive protein and Lp-PLA2—can serve as markers of a turned-on immune system, a warning sign that conditions are right for heart disease.

If a clot forms but narrows the artery by only 80 to 90 percent, it may cause chest pain that falls short of a full-blown heart attack. In time, the area of rupture may heal and shrink in size. This process can be repeated again and again.

In other words, plaque formation isn't simply a matter of sediment gathering on artery walls; it is a dynamic, inflammatory process. Cholesterol plays an important role in this process, but it is not the only—or necessarily the most important—marker of heart disease.

WHAT DOES PLAQUE RUPTURE FEEL LIKE?

Cardiovascular disease progresses slowly without fanfare for decades before it makes itself known, often in the form of a heart attack. Many people with heart disease have a vigilant warning system that alerts them to impending trouble. Typical symptoms of a narrowed artery include chest pain or pressure that is brought on by exercise or stress and relieved with rest.

Warning signs in women are often more difficult to interpret. Symptoms of heart disease in women tend not to be the typical ones experienced by men but, instead, can include shortness of breath or irregular heartbeats.

Sadly, for up to half of both men and women with serious cardiovascular disease, a defective warning system fails to alert them to impending doom. Their first symptom is a full-blown heart attack.

Heart attack victims often delay seeking medical help, frequently with fatal results. Most deaths from heart attacks occur in the first two hours after symptoms develop, yet studies have shown that many people wait four to six hours to get to an emergency room. Never ignore the warning signs of a heart attack. They include:

- Chest pain—an uncomfortable pressure, fullness, squeezing, or crushing feeling in the center of the chest that lasts two minutes or longer. Often this discomfort is described as "pressure" or "tightness" rather than pain.
- Severe pain that radiates to the shoulders, neck, arms, jaw, or top of the stomach.
- Shortness of breath.
- Sweating.
- Rapid or irregular pulse.
- Dizziness, fainting, or loss of consciousness.

Cardiologists can limit your damage from a heart attack and improve your chances of survival by opening up the blocked artery with balloons and stents. These treatments are most effective if delivered within the very first hours of a heart attack.

If the blood supply is not restored within three to six hours, most of the cells in that part of the heart muscles will die and be replaced by scar tissue. The take-home message is clear: If you experience the symptoms listed above, get emergency medical care without delay.

UNDERSTANDING THE ROLE OF CHOLESTEROL

Although cholesterol is far from the only trigger of heart disease, it certainly has emerged as a very key player. Literally tens of thousands of patients have participated in well-controlled medical studies irrefutably proving that treating cholesterol problems lowers the risk of heart attacks and saves lives. Still, some argue that cholesterol is not an important risk and offer up the following argument: If cholesterol is so important, why is it that so many heart attack victims have normal cholesterol, while others with high levels never go on to develop heart disease?

The answer lies in a more sophisticated understanding of the meaning of *normal cholesterol*. A desirable total cholesterol level is often described as 200 mg/dL or less, and it is certainly true that at least one-third of heart attacks occur in those with a total cholesterol level under 200 mg/dL. Many of these people who are glibly described as having a normal cholesterol value actually have very severe cholesterol problems, but these problems are not identifiable by a superficial glance at the test results. For example, some individuals have a low total cholesterol level yet far too little of the protective HDL cholesterol; others may have dangerous levels of other fats that are not typically measured.

Chapter 3 will describe the information available in a standard cholesterol profile, and chapter 4 will explore other tests that go beyond cholesterol in providing a comprehensive picture of your cardiovascular health.

TAKE THIS TO HEART

- Damage to the arteries from atherosclerosis often begins in childhood and young adulthood.
- Heart attacks are not caused by the passive buildup of cholesterol in the arteries, but from a complex and dynamic process in which inflammation plays a key role.
- A so-called normal total cholesterol level can mask severe risks that require further testing to uncover.

Chapter 3

Traditional Cholesterol Tests:
What They Tell You—and
What They Don't

Rachel was thirty-nine when she made her first appointment with me. She had recently had a cholesterol check with her gynecologist, and her total cholesterol was an admirable 125. Sounds good, but she was actually facing a serious cholesterol problem: Her good HDL cholesterol registered at only 18. (The optimal level for a woman is over 50.) Her gynecologist advised her not to worry about her low HDL, however, since her total cholesterol was so low. She felt reassured until a few weeks before her fortieth birthday, when she experienced an alarming sensation of chest pressure during exercise. An abnormal stress test prompted an angiogram that uncovered two arteries narrowed by 70 percent.

This serious finding occurred well before menopause in a woman who did not smoke, was not a diabetic, and had normal blood pressure. Was her low HDL a problem? Absolutely. Can a low level of total cholesterol hide other cholesterol problems that threaten your heart? Yes! The relationship between cholesterol and heart disease is more complicated than most people—and many doctors—appreciate.

CHOLESTEROL: TOO MUCH—OR TOO LITTLE— OF A GOOD THING

Cholesterol is vital for life: It keeps our cells strong and serves as the chemical backbone of many key hormones. The liver is where the magic happens, churning out the cholesterol needed to keep our bodies in balance. Unfortunately, in many people the levels of some kinds of cholesterol far exceed the minimum requirement. The human body, in its infinite wisdom, has a built-in control system that produces a good cholesterol to help mop up excesses of potentially dangerous excess LDL cholesterol.

In this chapter, we will explore the different types of cholesterol and learn that there is much more to consider than your total cholesterol number when assessing cardiac risk. Cholesterol is measured as milligrams per deciliter of blood (mg/dL), but for simplicity, it will be written in this book without the label.

A standard cholesterol profile includes a measurement of total cholesterol, LDL, HDL, and triglycerides. With so many variables to consider, how do you go about evaluating your risk?

Although most people focus on their total cholesterol level, this value is just the beginning. The total cholesterol is the grand total of many kinds of fats, a combination of "Lousy" LSL cholesterol, "Helpful" HDL cholesterol, and the triglyceride level divided by 5 (just to make things confusing).

You can imagine the paradox that this mixed bag presents. A rise in total cholesterol, for example, can actually be a good thing if it is caused solely by an elevation in HDL. Similarly, risk can soar with a drop in total cholesterol if the decline is based on a drop in HDL. Because of all the surprises that can be hidden inside the total cholesterol number, it is much more useful to evaluate each of the individual fats separately.

LDL is the most important cholesterol value to determine your risk of heart disease. LDL is the main ingredient in plaque that weakens arteries, leading to heart disease and stroke. The liver makes LDL cholesterol, and levels are determined by your genes, diet, and exercise habits. Diets rich in cholesterol, saturated fats, or trans fats will raise LDL cholesterol. To the chagrin of many health-conscious people, levels of LDL can still be high despite a healthy diet and exercise program if you were born with the wrong genes.

HDL is the good twin; the more HDL, the better. When it comes to gender, HDL is not an equal opportunity provider; women enjoy higher levels (50 to 55) compared with men (40 to 45). Risk increases in women when values drop under 50, and in men when levels fall below 40. HDL is made by the liver, with a production quota largely determined by your genetic inheritance. HDL can also be influenced, however, by your environment, including exercise, weight loss, supplements, and medication (see chapters 6 and 11).

HDL is beneficial because it is a chemical garbage truck, hauling away the lousy LDL from the arteries and depositing it back in the liver. HDL also acts as an antioxidant, keeping LDL in a form that cannot enter plaque as easily.

Ideally, LDL and HDL work together in balance. Too often, however, LDL production exceeds the body's demands for it, and the body has too little HDL on hand to clear away the excess. When this happens—particularly when levels of inflammation are high—the LDL cholesterol collects on the walls of the arteries.

Triglycerides are another category of fat used by the body as a source of energy. Triglycerides provide the fuel needed for active muscles, but, under conditions of overabundance, they are warehoused into fat cells. Interestingly, high triglyceride levels are linked to heart disease even more in women than men. Risk is especially high when elevated triglycerides are paired with low HDL.

Triglycerides are made in the liver, and levels are dramatically influenced by diet, especially simple carbohydrates (such as white bread, white potatoes, and white rice), alcohol, and saturated fat. I have seen wild variations in triglycerides based on even a single carbohydrate binge; values typically soar the day after a visit to the dessert bar. Diabetics also typically have high triglyceride levels that improve when sugar levels are brought under control.

SETTING CHOLESTEROL GOALS

What should your cholesterol levels be to lower your risk of heart attack? The Adult Treatment Panel (ATP) of the National Cholesterol Education Program has issued a set of guidelines for cholesterol management. (See the references in "Chapter Notes" to review the updated guidelines in detail.) The recommendations below are the goals I set for my own patients, which are more stringent than those listed in the ATP Guidelines. I generally aim for more aggressive goals because I believe they are associated with reduced risk compared with the ATP Guidelines.

Total Cholesterol

A total cholesterol level less than 200 is often considered ideal. For the reasons previously mentioned, however, many significant risks can be hidden inside a low total cholesterol level. In fact, one-third of those with heart disease have a total cholesterol less than 200, rendering this term a poor predictor of heart disease. For this reason, I advise my patients to disregard this number and focus on the component fat levels that make up the total.

KNOWING YOUR NUMBERS

Cholesterol is measured in milligrams per deciliter (mg/dL).

LDL Cholesterol

Under 70	Optimal for those with heart disease or diabetes
70–100	Optimal for those without heart disease or diabetes
100–129	Mildly elevated risk
130–159	Borderline high risk
160–189	High risk
190 and above	Very high risk

HDL Cholesterol

Over 60	Optimal
Under 50	Increased risk for women
Under 40	Increased risk for men

Triglycerides

Under 100	Optimal
100–150	Borderline elevated
150–199	Mildly elevated

| 200–499 | High |
| 500 and higher | Very high |

A full cholesterol profile should only be drawn after a full ten-hour fast (water and medication not included). Blood drawn with less than a ten-hour fast will not give reliable results as to triglycerides or LDL.

DO I NEED TO WORRY ABOUT LDL IF MY HDL IS HIGH?

While high HDL is desirable, it does not completely compensate for a high LDL. When discussing this issue with my patients, I ask them the following question: What does it take to stop your car? Answer: Good tires and good brakes. So, I continue, if your tires are in the best shape, does it still matter if your brakes are shot? Of course it does. Similarly, a desirable HDL cannot completely remove the risk of high LDL. Your goal is to consider LDL and HDL separately, and to optimize both.

How Low Should LDL Be?

Your LDL goals should be set based on your individual health challenges. Recent studies show that for high-risk individuals—defined as those with heart disease or diabetes—LDL levels well under 100 mg/dL are optimal. The PROVE-IT study (the acronym stands for "Pravastatin or Atorvastatin Evaluation and Infection Therapy") evaluated moderate versus intensive

LDL lowering in individuals with heart disease. In the moderate group, LDL was lowered to a level of 95; in the intensive group, it was pushed down to 62. The study showed that those with their LDL lowered to 62 had far fewer repeat heart attacks than those who saw it reduced to only 95.

The landmark Heart Protection Study, published in the British medical journal *The Lancet* in 2002, found that for high-risk individuals, a statin medication lowered the risk of heart problems even if the LDL level before treatment was under 100. People taking simvastatin had lower cholesterol and 24 percent fewer heart attacks compared with people in the control group.

These studies lend support to the concept that, for high-risk individuals, LDL values under 70 are ideal.

Those without a history of vascular disease or diabetes—who are, therefore, at lower risk—should optimally have an LDL value anywhere under 100.

Is there a risk of other side effects from driving LDL too low? This is an important, but unanswered question, currently under investigation.

Keeping Your HDL High

When it comes to HDL cholesterol, your goal is to raise the number as high as possible. I tell my patients to aim L—Lower for LDL and H—Higher for HDL. Raising HDL is usually more difficult than lowering LDL, but the good news is that small increases in HDL make a big impact on risk reduction. For each 1 mg/dL increase in HDL, men can expect up to a 2 percent decrease in heart attack risk; women enjoy a 3 percent lower risk.

The importance of high HDL was discovered with the

Framingham Heart Study, which involved thousands of people in Framingham, Massachusetts. Researchers found that among people with the same LDL, those with higher HDL had fewer heart attacks than those with lower HDL.

HDL levels tend to plummet in those with a high-carbohydrate diet, sedentary lifestyle, or diabetes, as well as among smokers. Part 2 of this book includes specific suggestions to raise HDL with natural treatments.

Don't Overlook Your Triglyceride Level

High triglyceride levels are an independent risk factor for heart disease, especially in women. Very high triglyceride levels (500 or more) can cause life-threatening inflammation of the pancreas.

A triglyceride test is part of a full cholesterol profile. Because your triglyceride level quickly responds to what you eat, it is essential that you fast for at least ten hours beforehand for reliable results.

A number of factors can increase triglyceride levels, including some drugs (steroids, beta-blockers, and estrogen), a high-carbohydrate diet, alcohol, a sedentary lifestyle, excess weight, and diabetes.

Among all the fat levels, triglycerides respond best to lifestyle changes, especially weight loss and exercise. Other factors that can lower triglyceride levels include a diet high in mono-unsaturated fat and low in saturated and trans fats, as well as the use of fibrates, niacin, and statins.

ARE YOU AT RISK?

I recommend regular cholesterol screening tests for all children and adults. Adults should be checked once a year, and more often if problems are uncovered. In addition to basic cholesterol testing, people at risk of heart disease also need further testing to identify other cardiovascular risk factors that go beyond cholesterol. Throughout this book, I will make different recommendations for people at risk of heart disease and stroke. There are several specific factors that define the at-risk patient (in addition to cholesterol problems that will be discussed in detail in chapter 4):

- **Family history.** This category includes anyone with a family member who has suffered a heart attack or stroke. Among those with family history, there are various degrees of risk: The closer the family member (parent or sibling rather than uncle or grandfather, for instance), the younger the family member at the time of the cardiac event (especially under fifty-five for men and under sixty-five for women), and the more family members with a history of disease, the higher the risk.
- **Diabetics.** A patient is considered diabetic if he or she has a fasting blood sugar rate of 126 mg/dL or greater.
- **Pre-diabetic.** A patient is considered pre-diabetic with a fasting blood sugar rate of 100 to 125.
- **High blood pressure.** A reading of 140/90 is classified as high blood pressure, or 130/80 if a person has diabetes.
- **Smoking.** Cigarette smokers are at much greater risk of heart disease than nonsmokers.

Other risk factors that contribute to cardiac risk include sedentary behavior, obesity, and the metabolic syndrome (see the box).

DO YOU HAVE METABOLIC SYNDROME?

I recognize metabolic syndrome as a significant cardiac risk factor. *Metabolic syndrome* is a stew of unfavorable ingredients; individually, none is as extreme as those listed in "Are You at Risk?", but when grouped together, they *double the risk* of heart disease. This syndrome is a colossal public health problem—affecting more than one in four adults.

Metabolic syndrome is diagnosed if three or more of the following conditions are present:

- Abdominal obesity—a waist measurement of more than 40 inches in men or 35 inches in women.
- Triglyceride levels greater than 150 mg/dL.
- HDL levels less than 40 mg/dL in men or less than 50 mg/dL in women.
- Borderline high blood pressure—more than 130/85.
- Borderline high blood sugar—above 100 mg/dL.

Lifestyle changes are the foundation of all prevention programs. Still, even with very determined effort, some patients cannot optimize their risk factors through lifestyle changes alone. In these cases, genetics likely account for the persistent problems. I often tell my conscientious patients who do everything right but can't get their cholesterol down naturally that they made one big mistake: They picked the wrong parents!

Fortunately, people with bad genes and a family history of heart disease *can* take steps to minimize their risk by identifying and addressing all of their potential risk factors. Available blood tests can warn you of existing cardiovascular disease, even when your traditional cholesterol screening doesn't. If you have some reason to be concerned about your cardiac health, these tests can possibly provide you with lifesaving information. The following chapter discusses various blood tests that will provide more information than basic cholesterol screening. Part 2 of this book will provide information on how to reduce any risk factors identified by the tests.

TAKE THIS TO HEART

- When assessing your cholesterol numbers, do not focus on your total cholesterol level; instead, consider your LDL and HDL numbers as separate risk factors. Strive for LDL below 100 (or below 70 if you have a history of heart disease or stroke or diabetes). Aim for HDL above 45 (men) or 55 (women).
- Elevated triglycerides are an independent risk factor for cardiovascular disease. The goal is to keep your triglyceride level under 100; a level of 100 to 150 is borderline elevated, but acceptable.
- People at risk of heart disease include those with a family history of heart disease, or a personal history of diabetes, high blood pressure, or smoking.
- The metabolic syndrome, consisting of a mixture of milder versions of the risk factors listed above, doubles the risk of heart disease.

Chapter 4

Digging Deeper: Beyond Cholesterol

To win the battle against cardiovascular disease, you need to first identify your opponents. Cholesterol is the best-known cardiac culprit, but remember that half of all heart attacks occur in people with normal cholesterol levels. You might never have heard about small, dense LDL particles or lipoprotein (a), but these factors can trigger a heart attack, even if your LDL and HDL numbers fall into the desirable range. In fact, most patients with an alarming family history of heart disease have fairly desirable cholesterol levels; only further testing for these additional risk markers identifies the root of their unhealthy inheritance.

Four of the most important tests—*ones that should be included in a comprehensive evaluation of anyone concerned about heart attack risk*—are high-sensitivity C-reactive protein (CRP), LDL particle size, Lp(a), and homocysteine. The results of these four core tests, paired with the routine cholesterol profile, create the detailed road map you need to develop an optimal prevention program.

Paradoxically, treatments resulting from these high-tech

tests are surprisingly low-tech, often including the use of over-the-counter supplements (such as niacin or fish oil) and lifestyle changes (cutting back on simple carbohydrates, for instance, and ramping up your exercise program).

I recommend these four tests for all of my patients at risk of heart attack, including people with a family history of cardiovascular disease and those with high blood pressure, diabetes, or elevated cholesterol. When determining a patient's cardiac risk, I rely on all four tests, in addition to a complete cholesterol profile, of course. Together, the data for all of these tests create a more complete story of the patient's condition than the results of one or two of the tests examined separately.

OVERCOMING BAD GENES

Three of the four tests described in this chapter—LDL particle size, Lp(a), and homocysteine—are heavily influenced by your genes. Measurement of these inherited markers often reveals extreme abnormalities that help us understand why heart disease is so common in certain families. Abnormalities in these tests explain many surprise heart attacks that strike people with normal cholesterol profiles.

Even if your test results indicate that you have inherited unhealthy values of these markers, however, your genes need not dictate your cardiovascular fate. Think of the level of these chemicals in your body as being adjusted by an internal thermostat. Your genes dictate the factory setting, so to speak, of your body's chemical thermostats. You will default to these presets unless steps are taken to adjust the settings, such as taking supplements or making lifestyle adjustments.

That's the good news: You can lower your Lp(a) level and improve your particle size using the treatments described in this book. Although many doctors may not be aware of them, the treatment outlines in this chapter and in part 2 of this book can go a long way toward helping you avoid a heart attack.

CRP: C-REACTIVE PROTEIN

High-sensitivity C-reactive protein (CRP) is a smoking gun indicating that a fight is going on somewhere in your body, a fight that can involve many combatants, including traumatic injury, cigarette smoke, bacteria, and inflamed arteries caused by heart disease. High levels of CRP help predict heart attacks, strokes, and sudden cardiac catastrophes. As a screening test for heart problems, CRP predicts equally well in men and women, smokers and nonsmokers, the elderly and middle-aged, and diabetics and nondiabetics. Most physicians are familiar with CRP testing, although it is not as widely used as I believe it should be.

Why Should You Be Tested for CRP?

Think of CRP as a kind of lens: If CRP is elevated, it magnifies the risk of other factors; if it's low, it reduces the risk. Recent studies show that even when cholesterol levels appear desirable, your risk of heart attack is increased if CRP is high. For example, if you have a borderline LDL level—perhaps just over 100—the presence of a high CRP argues for more aggressive treatment, while a low CRP might tip the balance in favor of less intensive therapy.

In January 2003, the American Heart Association and the Centers for Disease Control and Prevention issued recommendations for CRP testing. These guidelines recommend CRP testing for people with a moderate risk of heart disease. This group includes people over age fifty; those with high blood pressure, high cholesterol, or a family history of heart disease; and smokers. About 40 percent of adult Americans fall into this midlevel group.

What Do the CRP Test Results Mean?

Because a number of transient health problems can bump up CRP, I recommend that those with an abnormally high level have a repeat test at least one month later. By waiting at least a month before performing a second CRP test, the body has a chance to resolve any temporary problem that may have contributed to an elevated reading on the initial test. Infections and other inflammatory conditions (such as a flare-up of arthritis) can cause CRP to temporarily soar, reaching levels of 10 mg/L or higher. Again, CRP levels drop quickly once the source of the inflammation has passed. I use the lower of the two scores when considering cardiac risk. If the second test confirms an abnormal reading, I assume that CRP is truly high.

CRP levels typically range from 0 to 15 milligrams per liter (mg/L) of blood.

- CRP levels below 1 mg/L reduce the risk of heart disease.
- CRP levels from 1 to 3 mg/L are relatively neutral, neither increasing nor diminishing risk.
- CRP levels above 3 mg/L increase risk of heart disease.

A commonly encountered situation in which CRP levels are high is the metabolic syndrome, a constellation of symptoms typically consisting of excess weight distributed around the belly, high sugar levels, and high blood pressure. (Metabolic syndrome is discussed in chapter 3.) Belly fat, as opposed to weight distributed elsewhere, acts as a factory for chemicals that inflame the arteries and raise CRP. Losing this type of deep belly fat is especially helpful not only for taking a load off, but also for shutting down the toxic waste factory in your gut and reducing CRP.

CRP and Heart Disease: Consider the Evidence

Hundreds of studies support the role of CRP as an important tool for prediction of cardiovascular disease and heart attack. The following are a few key conclusions:

- Men with high levels of CRP are almost three times more likely to have heart attacks than men with low CRP levels. Researchers compared CRP levels of apparently healthy middle-aged men participating in the Physicians' Health Study, half of whom experienced a heart attack or stroke and half whom did not. They found that study participants with high CRP levels were 2.9 times more likely to have heart attacks than men with low levels, even after other risk factors were taken into account.

- CRP can be better than standard cholesterol testing at assessing cardiovascular risk among women. Dr. Paul Ridker, director of the Center for Cardiovascular Disease Prevention, and his colleagues at Brigham and Women's Hospital in Boston followed nearly twenty-eight thousand apparently healthy women for eight years. They found that the women's CRP levels directly related to their risk of heart attacks, strokes, and other cardiovascular events. In fact, CRP level proved to be a better predictor of cardiovascular disease than LDL levels. Women with the highest CRP levels were twice as likely as those with a high LDL level to have a heart attack or stroke or to die from heart disease. Surprisingly, women with a high CRP and low LDL were at greater risk than women with a low CRP and high LDL. Based on these results, even though your LDL may be reasonably well controlled (below 130 mg/dL), do not be lulled into a false sense of security if your CRP is high (above 3 mg/L).

- Men with elevated CRP levels are at increased risk of sudden cardiac death. A study of ninety-seven cases of sudden cardiac death among apparently healthy men in the Physicians' Health Study found that those men with the highest CRP levels were 2.8 times more likely to experience sudden cardiac death than those with the lowest CRP levels.

- CRP levels are associated with high blood pressure. A study of more than twenty thousand women ages forty-five and older found that those with the highest CRP levels were significantly more likely to develop high blood pressure than those with the lowest CRP levels.

Lowering Your CRP Level

If you need to lower your CRP level, the following steps can be helpful. (The suggestions are discussed in greater detail in part 2 of the book.)

- **Dietary changes.** Food choices proven to lower CRP include eating more omega-3 fatty acids (found in fish and fish oil supplements), avoiding trans fats, limiting high-glycemic foods, and increasing fiber intake. (For details on diet, see chapter 7.) Dr. Andrew Weil, the pioneering integrative physician, has summarized these dietary components into an anti-inflammatory diet described in his book *Healthy Aging*.

- **Weight loss.** A seventeen-pound weight loss over three months has been shown to lower CRP by 26 percent.
- **Exercise.** Pairing a low-fat diet with exercise (two and a half hours a week or more) lowered CRP 33 percent in men and 29 percent in women.
- **Brush and floss.** Inflamed gums raise CRP and, as a result, increase the chance of developing heart disease. That brushing and flossing your teeth can have an impact so far away, inside your heart, is a testament to the fact that the body is a delicate ecosystem.
- **Statins** lower CRP by up to 40 percent. The greatest benefit from statins appears to be in those with high LDL and high CRP. Zetia added to statins leads to further reduction in CRP and LDL. (See chapter 11.)
- **Fish oil** (1 to 4 grams daily) added to a statin reduces CRP much more than the statin alone. (See chapter 6.)
- **Aspirin** at doses of 160 milligrams or higher (one half of a full adult aspirin) lowers CRP and reduces cardiac risk. Those with the highest CRP before treatment benefit most.

THE SIZE OF LDL

Many people are aware that cholesterol can be broken down into HDL and LDL, but LDL itself can be further subdivided. The two basic forms of LDL are small, dense particles and large, fluffy ones. Everyone has a predominant LDL particle size that is largely dictated by their genetic inheritance. The size of your LDL has an enormous impact on the potential for damage to your arteries.

Think of your LDL level as a bathtub filled with balls. Your LDL score reflects the fill line on the side of the tub. Now comes the more advanced concept: That same level—say, 130 mg/dL—can be achieved by filling the tub either with thousands of small, dense marbles—or alternately, with far fewer light Ping-Pong balls.

When it comes to your cardiovascular health, having many small particles is much more dangerous than having fewer large particles, even though both LDL types measure the same in routine testing.

You might assume that large particles would be more prone to clog up the arteries than small ones, but the opposite is true! Imagine rolling balls of different sizes on a pavement with cracks. Small marbles would tend to get stuck in the cracks, while bigger balls would roll right over. Exactly the same thing happens with cholesterol particles: The small, dense ones get stuck in the arteries, while the large, fluffy ones tend to pass freely.

The other consideration is that the risk of plaque buildup is related to the total number of LDL particles. If your LDL of 130 mg/dL is mostly made up of small particles, you will have many more of them than another person with the same LDL level who has mostly large, fluffy particles. This fact helps explain why some people with apparently desirable LDL levels go on to have heart problems; they are at greater risk because their LDL is made up mostly of small, dense particles.

LDL particle size is often referred to as either Pattern A or Pattern B. *Pattern A* describes large, buoyant LDL particles, while *Pattern B* denotes small, dense LDL particles.

Small, dense LDL particles often keep company with low HDL, high triglycerides, and high sugar levels. In fact, having small, dense LDL is associated with an increased chance of developing diabetes in the future. The tendency to manufacture small, dense LDL has a strong genetic basis. A spot on chromosome 19 has been identified as the likely source of the body's code to produce the small form of LDL.

Do You Need an LDL Particle Size Test?

I recommend tests for LDL particle size and particle number as part of the initial workup for all patients at increased risk of heart disease. Those data greatly extend the scope of information available from the more typical measurement of LDL cholesterol alone. If undesirable values are found, I recommend repeating the test after appropriate therapy to determine the extent of improvement. This test is important even for people with total cholesterol in the normal range.

What Do the Test Results Mean?

Most LDL particle size measurements are performed by one of a handful of national laboratories, and each uses a different method. Although each of these national labs claims advantages over the other labs, no one method has been proven superior to the others. Reports typically include both a numerical description of the particle size and a classification as either the large Pattern A or the small Pattern B forms. The ideal situation is to have the fewest particles possible, with the predominant form consisting of the large Pattern A variety.

About 50 percent of men and 30 percent of premenopausal women with coronary heart disease have inherited the tendency to make small, dense LDL. Small LDL does appear more often in people who consume a high-carbohydrate diet, are overweight, and don't exercise.

LDL Particle Size and Heart Disease: Consider the Evidence

LDL particle size has become an important measure of cardiovascular health. Following are a few key findings:

- Small, dense LDL increases risk of cardiovascular disease, even among people with cholesterol in the normal range. People with small, dense LDL are three times more likely than those with large, buoyant LDL to have coronary artery disease, even if their total cholesterol is in the normal range. The risk doubles to six times for people with large numbers of these small LDL particles.
- High levels of small, dense LDL have been found to be an independent cardiac risk factor. Elevated levels of the smallest subclass of LDL have been shown to be an independent factor for cardiac disease in a four-year study of men with heart disease. Men with the smallest LDL particle had a sixfold faster buildup of plaque than those with large LDL particles.
- Women tend to have lower levels of small, dense LDL than men. Researchers at the Centers for Disease Control looked at blood samples from more than three thousand men and women in the Framingham Offspring Study. They found that premenopausal women tended to have larger LDL and HDL particles, although the differences tended to diminish with age.

Converting to a More Friendly LDL

Despite the genetic influences, it is possible to convert small, dense LDL into the larger, less risky forms. In my practice, I see many patients move from small LDL into the less risky large variety by making the simple lifestyle changes discussed in part 2. Here is a summary of the approaches I have found useful in my practice:

- Maintain a healthy weight. (For more information, see chapter 7.)
- Eat a diet low in simple sugars and high in heart-healthy monounsaturated fats. (For more information, see chapter 7.)
- Consume 1 to 4 grams of fish oil daily. Fish oil (combined EPA and DHA) has a potent effect in converting small to large LDL. (See chapter 6.)
- Exercise regularly. Exercise has been shown to decrease total cholesterol while also decreasing the concentrations of small, dense LDL particles. (See chapter 9.)
- If the above measures are not successful, addition of niacin or the prescription fibrates is very helpful in converting small, dense LDL into the more desirable large form. (See chapter 11.)

LP(A): "LDL WITH ATTITUDE"

Lipoprotein (a)—pronounced *lipoprotein little a*—is a complex combination of an LDL fat particle bound with a chemical that interferes with the body's ability to clot. This chemical sandwich of a fat and a blood-clotting stimulant is an obvious recipe for trouble. Concern over Lp(a) has been heightened by the observation that it is found in higher amounts in the plaques of patients with unstable heart symptoms compared with those whose disease is stable.

Lp(a) is an important independent risk factor and is present in up to 30 percent of people with heart disease. More striking, high Lp(a) is especially common in families plagued with early heart disease. African Americans are an exception because, for reasons that are not well understood, they tend to have higher levels of Lp(a) without the associated increase in risk. High levels of Lp(a) raise your risk of coronary artery disease up to 300 percent, even if your standard cholesterol numbers look good.

Do You Need an Lp(a) Test?

I recommend the Lp(a) test to all of my patients; elevated Lp(a) can be present in people with desirable LDL and HDL levels. Lp(a) is a common problem in families with a striking history of early heart disease. Because Lp(a) is not often included in the panel of routine blood tests, most people who have this problem are never identified.

In the event of borderline or elevated readings, I recommend follow-up testing to assess the response to treatment.

What Do the Test Results Mean?

An Lp(a) level below 30 mg/dL is desirable. Levels above 30 mg/dL are associated with an increased risk of cardiovascular disease.

Lp(a) and Heart Disease: Consider the Evidence

Based on a growing body of science, the links among high Lp(a), heart attacks, and strokes are now clear. Here are some of the more notable findings:

- Elevated Lp(a) is an established independent risk factor for cardiovascular disease. It is linked to increased risk for heart attack, stroke, and coronary artery disease, among other issues.
- People with the highest Lp(a) levels are 1.5 times more likely to experience coronary heart disease than those with the lowest levels. French researchers investigated Lp(a) as a cardiovascular risk factor in more than nine thousand apparently healthy men. A high Lp(a) level was determined to be a risk factor for future heart pain, heart attack, and death from heart disease.
- Elevated Lp(a) is an independent predictor of stroke and death from vascular disease. Researchers at the Center for Cardiovascular Disease Prevention and Intervention in Dallas studied the role of Lp(a) on the cardiovascular health of almost six thousand men and women ages sixty-five and older. They divided the subjects into five groups based on their Lp(a) levels at the start of the seven-year study. They found that men in the highest Lp(a) group had three times the risk of stroke and almost three times the risk of death from a vascular event compared with those in the lowest group.
- Elevated Lp(a) is an excellent predictor of developing heart symptoms in healthy men, particularly when combined with a high LDL level. Researchers with the Physicians' Health Study looked at the Lp(a) levels of four

hundred men, half of whom developed heart pain and half of whom remained healthy over a five-year period. The risk of developing heart pain was four times greater in men with the highest Lp(a) levels, and twelve times higher in men with high Lp(a) and high LDL cholesterol.

Lowering Your Lp(a) Level

The amount of Lp(a) in your blood is mostly determined by your genes. Lp(a) is unusual in that, unlike other risk factors, levels don't respond to diet and exercise. Still, you can lower your level with the following over-the-counter supplements and food:

- Niacin (whether over the counter or by prescription) is the most effective agent currently available to lower Lp(a). A dose of 500 to 2,000 milligrams daily has been shown to slash levels by one-third. (For more information, see chapter 6.)
- L-carnitine helps lower Lp(a) levels, typically by 8 percent. Take 1 gram twice a day. (Again, see chapter 6.)
- Walnuts—about ten per day—can lower Lp(a) by up to 6 percent.

KEEP YOUR EYE ON LP-PLA2

Lp-PLA2 is a new blood test that promises to become an important tool for cardiac risk assessment. Lp-PLA2 is a chemical that inflames blood vessels, provoking vascular eruptions that cause heart attacks. CRP is also a measure of inflammation, but it does not differentiate between inflammation of blood vessels and inflammation from other sources, such as arthritis, infections, and so forth. Lp-PLA2, on other hand, is a more specific marker of diseased arteries than CRP. Risk of heart attack rises sharply when Lp-PLA2 levels exceed 223 ng/ml in blood.

Even when you think you can rest assured because your cholesterol level is low, an elevated Lp-PLA2 is a red flag, associated with twice the risk of those with low Lp-PLA2. High levels of both Lp-PLA2 and CRP are even more worrisome; this combination is associated with four times the risk of heart disease compared with those who have low levels of both.

Studies have shown that Lp-PLA2 levels can be reduced through statin and fenofibrate therapy. (See chapter 11 for information on drug treatments.) One potential application of Lp-PLA2 is to improve detection and guide treatment of inflamed arteries better than currently possible with CRP testing.

HOMOCYSTEINE

Homocysteine is an amino acid formed when the body breaks down dietary protein, especially protein from animal sources. When the system works as it should, the body completely converts methionine into cysteine, using the B vitamins—particularly folic acid and vitamins B_6 and B_{12}—to complete the metabolic process. However, when the body lacks the required levels of B vitamins, the process cannot be completed, so homocysteine levels rise. High homocysteine levels are linked to a higher risk of heart disease and stroke.

The reason for this relationship is not clear. Controversy continues as to whether homocysteine itself is damaging to the blood vessels, or if it is only a marker of other problems. There are a number of theories about how homocysteine contributes to heart disease. It may damage the delicate lining of blood vessels, stimulate the formation of blood clots, or generate toxic free radicals. Elevated homocysteine levels have also been linked to Alzheimer's disease, dementia, and Parkinson's disease.

Homocysteine levels drop considerably after treatment with high doses of folic acid, B_6, and B_{12}. However, high-dose vitamin treatment has been called into question recently, after large studies of people with known heart disease showed no benefit, and even the possibility of harm. These results discourage treatment with high-dose folic acid (more than 400 mcg), although daily treatment with a multivitamin that contains 400 mcg may still be appropriate. A great deal more research is needed in this area, including more research of treatment in people without heart disease, as well as in those with markedly elevated homocysteine levels.

Do You Need a Homocysteine Test?

Although the ideal treatment of abnormal homocysteine has been called into question, the fact remains that elevated homocysteine identifies people at increased risk for heart disease and stroke. For that reason, I still include a test for homocysteine as part of my initial evaluation.

What Do the Test Results Mean?

Homocysteine can be found at low levels in the blood of healthy people, but high levels indicate increased risk of cardiovascular disease.

- Homocysteine levels below 10 micromoles per liter of blood are optimal.
- Levels of 10 to 14 micromoles are mildly elevated.
- Levels above 14 micromoles are associated with increased risk of heart disease and stroke.

Homocysteine and Heart Disease: Consider the Evidence

Since the mid-1980s, hundreds of studies have reported a link between high levels of homocysteine and heart disease. Here are a few key ones:

- Elevated homocysteine levels are directly linked to heart attack risk. In 1992, the Physicians' Health Study of fifteen thousand participating doctors found that those who had a homocysteine level of 15 or more were three times as likely to have a heart attack as those with lower levels, even after taking other risk factors into account. Those with a level of 12 were twice as likely to have a heart attack.
- Lowering homocysteine with high doses of folic acid (800 mcg or greater), B_6, and B_{12} showed no benefit in reducing the risk of heart attacks in those with vascular disease. These trials raise questions as to whether homocysteine is a marker for disease rather than a root cause. Another possibility is that high doses of folic acid, B_6, and B_{12} might cause some unknown harm that counters the benefit of lowering homocysteine. More studies are needed in this area.
- High homocysteine levels are associated with increased risk of cardiovascular death. The Homocysteine and Progression of Atherosclerosis Study looked at whether

coronary heart disease and cerebrovascular disease progressed more rapidly in people with high homocysteine levels. After adjusting for age, smoking, hypertension, diabetes, and cholesterol, it was found that each 1-micromole increase in homocysteine level resulted in a 5.6 percent increased risk of death from cardiovascular disease in a three-year period.

Lowering Your Homocysteine Level

Based on recent studies, I no longer routinely recommend high-dose folic acid (more than 400 mcg daily) for patients with elevated homocysteine levels. Instead, I advise taking a multivitamin that contains 400 mcg of folic acid, in addition to eating foods rich in folic acid, including vegetables (lettuce, cabbage, asparagus), fruit (oranges, strawberries, melons), and whole grains.

In addition, I recommend that my patients reduce their consumption of animal products, especially meat and dairy. Dr. David DeRose of the Lifestyle Center of America lowered the homocysteine levels of forty men and women in a one-week study using diet alone. By completely avoiding all animal products, caffeine, and alcohol, the study participants reduced their homocysteine levels by an average of 13 percent in just seven days.

Lastly, psychological stress can raise homocysteine levels. Stress-reduction techniques may be useful to lower levels and reduce risk. (For more information on stress reduction, see chapter 8.)

HOW OFTEN SHOULD YOU BE TESTED FOR THESE NEW RISK MARKERS?

All of these tests should be done once, as part of a comprehensive exam for at-risk patients. After that, the CRP test and a routine cholesterol profile should be repeated as part of a yearly physical. Your LDL particle size, Lp(a), and homocysteine levels do not need to be checked as frequently because the results of these tests vary less over time.

When initial tests uncover abnormalities that require treatment, it is important that you be retested to monitor the effectiveness of your therapy, but once you reach desirable levels you can retest less frequently. The beauty of this approach is that success—or the need for more intensive treatment—is not a matter of speculation but, instead, clearly measurable.

If you have reason to believe you are at increased risk of heart disease, consider a consultation with a prevention specialist—a preventive cardiologist, or a prevention-focused internist or family physician. Look for someone who is familiar with these advanced risk factor tests and how to appropriately act on the results. Unless your physician has experience evaluating the results of these tests, you will not likely achieve the maximum benefit from them. Fortunately, many insurance companies cover the costs of these core tests.

In addition to the blood tests described in this chapter, your doctor may recommend a stress test or calcium heart scan. These tests are described in detail in the following chapter.

TAKE THIS TO HEART

Know your C-reactive protein (CRP) level. A level below 1 mg/L reduces your risk of heart disease. A level of 1 to 3 mg/L has no major impact on risk, while one above 3 mg/L increases your risk of heart disease—even with a desirable cholesterol level. You can lower your CRP level by:

- Consuming more fish, avoiding trans fats, and eating low-glycemic and high-fiber foods; see chapter 7.
- Taking fish oil; see chapter 6.
- Losing weight, if needed; see chapter 7.
- Getting regular aerobic exercise; see chapter 9.
- Brushing and flossing your teeth.
- Taking statins; see chapter 11.
- Taking aspirin at doses of 160 to 325 milligrams daily; see chapter 11.

Know your LDL particle size. You may have a cholesterol problem even if your standard profile appears desirable. Large, fluffy LDL (Pattern A) is optimal. Small, dense LDL (Pattern B) is less desirable. You can convert LDL from Pattern B to Pattern A by:

- Losing weight, if needed; see chapter 7.
- Restricting simple sugars; see chapter 7.
- Getting regular aerobic exercise; see chapter 9.
- Taking fish oil; see chapter 6.
- Taking niacin; see chapters 6 and 11.
- Taking fibrates; see chapter 11.

Know your Lp(a) level. Below 30 mg/dL is desirable, whereas a level above 30 mg/dL indicates increased risk. You can lower Lp(a) by:

- Taking niacin; see chapters 6 and 11.
- Taking L-carnitine; see chapter 6.
- Eating ten walnuts daily.

Know your homocysteine level. Below 10 micromoles/L is desirable. A level of 10 to 14 micromoles/L indicates a mildly elevated risk, while readings above 14 micromoles/L denote higher risk. You can lower your homocysteine by:

- Taking a multivitamin containing 400 micrograms of folic acid.
- Limiting red meat; see chapter 7.
- Reducing stress; see chapter 8.

Chapter 5

―◆◆◆―

What You Can Learn from Heart Scans and Stress Tests

My patients often ask me, "Do I need one of those heart scans I heard about?" You may be wondering the same thing; it's hard to turn on the radio or pick up a newspaper these days without being bombarded by advertisements from medical facilities offering lifesaving, quick, and painless heart scans. Inevitably, the person featured in the ad learned about a life-threatening coronary blockage that had not been detected by basic cholesterol screening. Choices now include calcium scans as well as the new sixty-four-slice CT scans.

After hearing these ads, you may wonder: Should you have a heart scan? Should you do it on your own or talk to your doctor about it first? The answers are not always clear-cut.

I believe that the blood tests described in the previous chapter are far more important than heart scans as screening tests. The blood tests allow you to evaluate for the actual *causes* of heart disease, as opposed to the imaging tests that track disease that has already developed. That being said, the allure of taking a sneak peek inside your heart is hard to resist. This chapter will review some of the most common imaging choices, so that you can discuss them with your doctor and decide which tests you need, and which you don't.

A TALE OF TWO PATIENTS

Two patients, Richard and Steve, came to see me after having undergone heart scans for coronary calcium. Neither had symptoms of heart disease or suffered from poor health, but both felt vulnerable because of a family history of heart disease, so they decided to have the tests done on their own.

There the similarities ended. When the results came in, Richard learned that he had a very high calcium score. He went on to have a shockingly abnormal stress test that led to a heart procedure confirming severe narrowing in all of the major arteries in his heart. Because his condition was so advanced, he needed coronary bypass surgery. Ten years later, Richard continues to do well, and he credits his heart scan with the early detection of a serious cardiac problem.

Steve's heart scan was entirely different. He learned that he had no appreciable calcium buildup in his arteries; his calcium score was 0. Given the glowing test result, he felt that he was in the clear and never followed up with his doctor. Unfortunately, nine months later, Steve suffered several bouts of severe chest pain. He saw a cardiologist, who opened up a critical narrowing in the key artery that supplies blood to the front of the heart. Steve's favorable calcium scan result gave him a false—and potentially dangerous—sense of security.

Richard and Steve are two patients who highlight the dilemma of coronary calcium scanning: Early detection can save lives, but a false sense of security can be dangerous. A patient at risk of heart disease should not independently obtain a heart scan and/or rely on a low calcium score as evidence of a clean bill of health.

CORONARY CALCIUM SCANS

These scans go by several names, including ultrafast CT, heart scans, and coronary calcium scans. All are variations on computed tomography (CT) scans, technology that has been used to noninvasively peer inside the body for more than twenty years. Image quality has improved as technology has advanced, but the main approach is the same. Areas of diseased arteries in the heart often (but not always) contain flecks of calcium. The scans detect very small amounts of calcium in the arteries, which are most often (but not always) part of the plaque.

Calcium in diseased arteries shows up as white spots on an otherwise dark image of the heart. A computer program measures the brightness and area of the white spots in the coronary arteries and calculates a total calcium score. The higher your calcium score, the more plaque is present in your arteries.

Interpretations of heart scans typically include not only the total calcium score, but also a number or percentile rank that describes how your score stacks up against other men or women of similar age. For example, a rank of 50 percent means that half of the people your age and gender have higher calcium scores than yours, and half have lower. Because the percentile rank takes into account your age and gender, it is generally considered more useful than the uncorrected total score. The optimal result is to be under the 50th percentile—and the lower, the better. Generally, scores over the 75th percentile are considered especially high risk.

Coronary Calcium Scans: Not a Perfect Predictor

Coronary calcium scans are not an absolute predictor of heart disease. It is possible to have soft plaque: diseased arteries with soft, cholesterol-laden buildups that do not contain calcium. This is more likely to happen in younger men and women. Just as my patient Steve experienced cardiac symptoms even though his calcium score was 0, these soft plaques can go on to cause chest pain and heart attacks, all without a trace of calcium showing up on the scan.

A study evaluating coronary calcium scores in the context of traditional risk factors was published in the *Journal of the American Medical Association* (*JAMA*) in 2004. The researchers found that a calcium score of 0 did not mean that participants were free of cardiac risk; in fact, seven of seventy-five people (9 percent) with a calcium score of 0 but a high risk of heart disease based on other risk factors went on to suffer a heart attack or cardiac death. So did 7 of 195 people (4 percent) with a 0 calcium score and fewer risk factors.

Coronary Calcium Scans Can't Replace Angiograms

Some patients mistakenly consider coronary calcium scans to be a substitute for an angiogram. An angiogram, also known as heart catheterization, is an invasive procedure in which a tube is placed into an artery in your body; dye is then injected into the heart to check for narrowed or blocked arteries. This test is the gold standard for finding blocked arteries and deciding if a procedure to open up the artery (an angioplasty or stent) is needed. Angiograms are far too invasive to be used as a screening test for the public; they carry a small but significant risk of causing a stroke or heart attack. Unfortunately, however, coronary calcium tests cannot determine if an artery is narrowed. An artery could be 20 percent or 99 percent narrowed and contain the same amount of calcium.

I sometimes explain this confusing idea to patients by likening a coronary calcium scan to a rust meter checking for blockage in the pipes at your house. Over time, household pipes can become rusty and corroded, and at some point a few may become narrowed or blocked. If you directed the rust meter at your pipes, you would get various rust readings. A high reading for rust could indicate wear and tear, but it does not prove that the pipe is narrowed and needs to be snaked out. Other kinds of tests would be needed to check the flow of water through the pipe. In the same way, coronary calcium scans may detect rust in the arteries, but they do not assess blood flow.

Coronary Calcium Scans Can Help Determine Risk

Although not a replacement for an angiogram, a heart scan can provide some very useful information about your heart health. As part of a study published in the journal *Circulation* in 2003, researchers from the University of Illinois collected coronary calcium scores from more than eighty-eight hundred adults with no cardiac symptoms. Patients were followed for more than three years, and calcium scores were studied in relation to their outcome. Men with the highest calcium scores (the 75th percentile or greater) were more than twice as likely to have a heart attack or die, compared with men with lower percentile rankings of coronary calcium. In women, percentile scores were not linked to heart attacks or death, but did help predict future need for angioplasty or coronary bypass procedures.

I support the use of calcium scores in the assessment of

people whose risk is in the gray zone—those who have some risk factors but not enough to put them in a high-risk category. A high coronary calcium score in this group could tip the balance in favor of more aggressive treatment of risk factors, while a low score could justify less intensive treatment. This approach is supported by a study from the 2004 *Journal of the American Medical Association,* in which those thought to benefit the most from coronary calcium scans were those with only a few milder risk factors for whom treatment decisions can be difficult. In this middle group, a total calcium score of better than 300 predicted a higher risk of heart problems.

Do you fall in this intermediate risk group? Risk assessment in the *JAMA* study was determined by the Framingham risk score, a measure that emerged from the landmark Framingham Heart Study. Investigators found the scan to be most helpful in the group with a 10 to 20 percent ten-year risk of heart disease based on this score. To calculate your own Framingham score, you must know your blood pressure and cholesterol values. Given this information, fill in your values at the following Web site: http://hp2010.nhlbihin.net/atpiii/calculator.asp.

For example, a fifty-five-year-old man with total cholesterol of 200 and an HDL of 40 who is treated for blood pressure with a recent reading of 145 systolic would have a Framingham risk score of 11 percent, putting him in the intermediate-risk category.

On the other hand, people considered to be at very low or very high risk on the basis of their history, cholesterol, and blood pressure did not stand to benefit as much from the scan, because they either clearly needed treatment or clearly were at low risk. In other words, I don't recommend coronary calcium scans for high-risk patients—who need treatment regardless of their calcium scores—or for low-risk patients, who do not need treatment regardless of their scores.

Coronary Calcium Scans Can Be Powerful Motivators

In my experience, patients often respond to the visual results of their coronary calcium scan—a picture showing the white clumps of calcium collected inside their arteries—far more dramatically than the more abstract concept of risk factors. Concern generated from the scan can motivate people to make lifestyle changes they might otherwise not be inclined to make. For those who order the scan on their own, without a doctor's prescription, an abnormal result may serve as the wake-up call that prompts a much-needed doctor's visit.

I am concerned, however, by the individuals who have significant cardiac risk factors but calcium scores of 0. In such cases, people often feel a false sense of security, and they may feel immune to their other risks and justified in not making necessary lifestyle changes.

Moving Closer to a Noninvasive Angiogram: The New Sixty-Four-Slice CT Scans

Recently released imaging equipment can take sixty-four simultaneous pictures—visual slices—of the heart. The resulting image quality is far beyond that seen with previous generations of eight- and sixteen-slice scanners. The sixty-four-slice scans now allow unprecedented detail of the inside of the artery as well as actual measurement of the presence and amount of narrowing, with results very similar to those obtained with the more invasive traditional angiogram. Such measurements are not possible with coronary calcium scans.

The accuracy of sixty-four-slice CT scans was compared with the traditional angiograms of the heart in two studies published in 2005. For identification of patients with a significant narrowing (more than 50 percent), the studies showed a sensitivity of 95 to 100 percent, and a specificity of 90 to 92 percent. Drawbacks of the sixty-four-slice scanner include the need to inject dye through an intravenous line (coronary calcium scans alone do not require dye); also the radiation dose is several times that of a coronary calcium scan and more than an invasive heart catheterization.

Do You Need a Heart Scan?

I strongly recommend that you talk to your doctor to decide if you would benefit from having either a coronary calcium scan or a sixty-four-slice CT scan. On the one hand, it can be argued that there is nothing to lose by performing the tests, and that knowledge is power. On the other, every test has a potential for harm; in this case, it could create either a false sense of security or abnormal results, prompting unnecessary invasive follow-up testing.

In my own practice, I favor testing for treatable risk factors with the blood studies mentioned in chapters 3 and 4 over the widespread use of scans. The advantage of emphasizing blood studies, paired with other risk factors (family history, diabetes, pre-diabetes, and high blood pressure), is that they allow me to examine the causes of any problems, along with identifying the custom treatment needed for each patient. If I see a patient with a strong family history of heart disease or one with a significant problem in the blood tests previously discussed, my plan is to aggressively treat all of the abnormalities identified.

I don't order a scan in such cases because regardless of its results, I would still advise intensive prevention efforts.

I do sometimes order a coronary calcium scan for people at intermediate risk; this scan may help me decide how aggressively to pursue treatment. I also consider a scan for those individuals who are in serious need of intensive lifestyle changes, but don't have the motivation. I do so hoping that a positive scan will spur them into action.

I am impressed with early data demonstrating a high degree of accuracy with the sixty-four-slice scanner compared with the invasive angiogram. Although it is unlikely to become a routine screening tool, given the radiation exposure and expense involved, I believe it will play an important role for selected patients. I have used the sixty-four-slice CT as a follow-up exam in intermediate-risk patients who have a mildly abnormal stress test. Since mildly abnormal stress tests often represent false alarms, I prefer going with a noninvasive test, such as the sixty-four-slice CT, as opposed to the usual invasive angiogram when further evaluation is needed. Conversely, in patients with very abnormal stress test results, I recommend proceeding directly to the traditional angiogram, since the likelihood of significant disease is high.

STRESS TESTS

A stress test is intended to give your heart a sort of test drive. This is important because—just as when you're sizing up a car on the lot before you buy it—you can't completely assess the inner workings of your heart without seeing how it responds when running at full throttle. The heart might appear to function normally at rest, but have hidden blockages that can only be revealed when under stress.

Stress tests are most often used for those with symptoms of chest pain or shortness of breath where the diagnosis of a heart condition is not clear. In other cases, a stress test might be ordered to evaluate for a hidden heart condition in sedentary people about to embark on an exercise program. There is another, seemingly paradoxical time when stress tests are used: to determine the impact on heart function from a borderline narrowing found on an angiogram. In this case, the stress test is ordered after the more invasive angiogram.

The stress test procedure involves monitoring the heart for signs of strain during gradually increasing exercise on either a treadmill or a stationary bicycle.

The EKG Stress Test

As you exercise, the electrical signature of your heartbeat is analyzed for abnormalities. Stress within narrowed arteries shows up as a sagging of part of the electrical signal. The problem with the EKG stress test is that it is well known to create many false alarms, especially in women. In other cases, the EKG stress test fails to detect important blockages, especially when only one artery is blocked. The EKG stress test misses as many as three out of ten people who have one severely diseased artery.

Flawed as it is, this test remains valuable in screening very low-risk individuals. I seldom use the EKG stress test alone in my practice; most often I combine it with either ultrasound (stress echocardiogram) or, less often, stress nuclear testing.

The Echocardiogram Stress Test

During this stress test, your doctor places an ultrasound "microphone" on your chest. The device transmits high-frequency sound waves similar to those used by a submarine's sonar. The sound waves bounce off the heart, providing a moving image of its beating. This technique examines your heart millimeter by millimeter, checking for motion in the main pumping chamber (left ventricle). Images of the heart are taken before and after exercise. The normal response is for the heart to become more vigorous after exercise. If, instead, part of the heart becomes weaker after exercise, plaque buildup in the arteries is suspected in the area that is not beating as expected. (The image shows the heart muscle, not the arteries, but it is possible to infer the condition of the arteries from the performance of the heart.) In general, this test detects up to 90 percent of individuals with severe heart disease (as opposed to approximately 70 percent with the EKG stress test). According to an article published in the *American Journal of Cardiology* in 2005, the echocardiogram stress test often identified problems missed by the EKG stress test alone; among those who went on to have a heart problem despite a normal EKG stress test, 60 percent had abnormalities detected on the echocardiogram stress test.

A Canadian study that focused on women experiencing chest pain reported similar results. According to a study published in the *Canadian Journal of Cardiology* in 2005, echocardiogram stress tests were more definitive and accurate than electrocardiogram stress tests.

The Nuclear Stress Test

During this stress test, images of your heart are taken after a small amount of a radioactive isotope is injected into your bloodstream. Pictures of the heart are then taken with a specialized camera that records signals from the radioactive isotope. Differences in the pictures between rest and exercise suggest lack of blood flow caused by a diseased artery.

Do You Need a Stress Test?

Stress tests are recommended for most people with risk factors for cardiovascular disease. In general, I recommend stress tests for patients over age forty who have significant risk factors for heart disease, including a family history of heart disease, or a personal history of diabetes, high blood pressure, or a cholesterol problem (as revealed in either the standard cholesterol tests or the new blood tests described in chapter 4). I also recommend stress tests for people over forty who have been fairly inactive and plan on starting a new exercise program. These emerging exercisers should have the test done prior to beginning their program to be on the lookout for serious problems that could place them at risk during vigorous activity. In general, the more risk factors you have, the more useful these tests can be in determining whether or not you have a cardiovascular problem.

While the EKG stress test is the most commonly available stress test, evidence suggests that stress tests that add some form of imaging of the heart—either echocardiogram or nuclear imaging—add substantially to the accuracy and reliability of the test results.

Bottom line: If you are over forty and have risk factors for heart disease or are about to start a new exercise program, talk to your doctor about arranging a stress test with either echocardiography or nuclear imaging.

TAKE THIS TO HEART

- Coronary calcium scans measure the amount of calcium deposited in the lining of the arteries, an indication of arterial plaque. The scans cannot determine if your artery is narrowed or blocked. Coronary calcium scores help predict the likelihood of heart disease, but are most useful in those at intermediate risk.

- Sixty-four-slice CT scans are the best noninvasive tool to examine the inside of your arteries and check for blockages. I believe this test is an ideal exam in selected patients who might otherwise be referred for an invasive angiogram (including those with mildly abnormal stress tests), but its cost and radiation exposure limit its widespread use as a screening tool.

- Before you make an appointment for any kind of heart scan, schedule a visit with a prevention-focused professional for a full workup, including the blood tests described in the previous chapters. These blood tests, paired with knowledge of your medical history, are the best way to identify and treat the root causes of heart disease.

- For those with significant risk factors determined from medical history and blood tests (the standard cholesterol profile, as well as the newer tests described in chapter 4), I recommend a stress test to check for evidence of severely diseased arteries.

- Stress tests that add pictures of the heart with either ultrasound (echocardiography) or nuclear imaging (thallium or technetium) are much more accurate than EKG stress tests at predicting cardiovascular disease.

PART 2

Take Action

Chapter 6

Supplements for a Healthy Heart

A seventy-three-year-old man recently traveled cross-country to see me for help with his dilemma. He had undergone coronary bypass surgery ten years before, but was vehemently opposed to taking prescription medications. He was careful with his diet and exercised regularly, but his LDL cholesterol was still too high: 167 (his minimum goal was under 100). I prescribed plant sterols—a nutritional supplement available at most health food stores—and recommended dietary changes. Within two months, his LDL cholesterol had dropped to 89. He accomplished the goal of lowering his LDL without relying on prescription drugs.

Another patient, a fifty-four-year-old man with a strong family history of heart disease, experienced similar success—as long as he stayed with his program. For several months, he followed a diet high in soy, plant sterols, fruits, and vegetables, because he wanted to avoid prescription medication. His LDL cholesterol fell from 147 to 112, and his C-reactive protein level plummeted from 12 to 0.2 (the optimal level is less than 1.0). The success of his diet caused him to get overconfident, however, and when he started to let his diet slip, his cholesterol and CRP levels crept back up, forcing him to acknowledge the importance of sticking with the diet.

I know from firsthand experience with thousands of patients that supplements can play a major role in lowering cholesterol. I am not against prescription medications in any way; for many, I believe they are lifesavers. That being said, I don't think prescriptions are needed for everyone with a cholesterol problem, and I believe there has to be room for flexibility based on the condition and the patient's own preferences. I believe in a goal-oriented approach. If we can achieve the cholesterol goals with nutrition, lifestyle, and supplements, great. However, when goals are not met with these approaches alone, it is time to move on to prescription medication. In people at high risk of heart disease or those with very severe cholesterol problems, I am inclined to start earlier with medication.

Many physicians overlook the use of supplements because they are not familiar with them. The use of supplements is generally not taught in medical school or included in medical training. In addition, it is far less likely that a sales representative from a supplement distributor will appear in a doctor's office than a representative from a pharmaceutical company.

I know that choosing supplements can be bewildering. In this chapter, we will focus on the key supplements that can make a major difference in your heart health.

The top heart-healthy supplements include (in order of importance):

- **Fish oil.** This anti-inflammatory nutritional supplement lowers the risk of heart disease and reduces triglycerides. I recommend it to all my patients.
- **Niacin.** This is the most effective agent available to raise

HDL. It also lowers LDL; converts dangerous small, dense LDL into the favorable large, fluffy form; and lowers triglycerides. In addition, it is the most potent agent available to reduce Lp(a).

- **Red yeast rice.** This is the best over-the-counter supplement to lower LDL cholesterol.
- **Stanols and sterols.** These are the second most powerful supplements to lower LDL cholesterol, and they have the fewest side effects.
- **Coenzyme Q10 (CoQ10).** This supplement helps replace key nutrients lost by people taking statins; it also helps control hypertension and treat heart failure.
- **Carnitine (L-carnitine).** This supplement helps lower Lp(a) levels.
- **Vitamin D.** This supplement lowers blood pressure and could reduce your risk of heart disease, especially in the winter months.

Please do not rush to your health food store and pick up all of these supplements. Just like medicine, supplements should be carefully chosen based on your individual needs, factoring in your diet, lifestyle, risk factors, and test results as outlined in part 1. I also recommend that people be guided by a health professional before taking any supplements: Some of them, even those purchased over the counter, require laboratory monitoring for safety and could interact with prescription medication.

WHICH SUPPLEMENTS DO YOU NEED?

If your LDL is high:

- Niacin
- Red yeast rice
- Stanols and sterol

If your HDL is low:

- Niacin

If your triglycerides are high:

- Fish oil
- Niacin

Is your Lp(a) is high:

- Niacin
- L-carnitine

If you take prescription statins or red yeast rice:

- Coenzyme Q10

If you have little exposure to the sun:

- Vitamin D

FISH OIL

Comparing Fish Oil and Prescription Medications

Fish oil is less potent than prescription fibrates, a prescription drug most often used to lower triglycerides, but it is the most effective over-the-counter product for this purpose. Omacor, a prescription omega-3 drug, is also available; this is a more concentrated form of omega-3 than over-the-counter supplements, but it is otherwise similar. (Omacor can be cheaper than taking fish oil supplements for some people, depending on their drug plan.) Prescription medications are discussed in chapter 11.

How It Works

Fish oil is the best source of omega-3 fatty acids. (Little-known fact: Fish do not manufacture omega-3 "fish oil"; the omega-3 fatty acids found in fish actually originate in microscopic algae and plankton, which are then eaten and concentrated in fish.) Fish oils contain large amounts of two omega-3 fatty acids, eicosapentaenoic acid (EPA) and docosahexaenoic acid (DHA). EPA and DHA have a wide range of health-promoting properties, most notably a potent anti-inflammatory effect. Fish oil is perhaps the most useful of all supplements for heart health, as well as other health concerns. These are some of its benefits for heart health:

- It lowers triglyceride levels.
- It converts small, dense LDL into the more favorable fluffy form.
- It lowers blood pressure (especially DHA).
- It reduces irregular heartbeat.

- It prevents sudden death after a heart attack.
- It serves as a mild blood thinner.

Fish oil also offers benefits for general health, including the following:

- It reduces arthritis pain.
- It may be helpful for certain neurological conditions, including attention deficit disorders and autism.

Using Fish Oil

Take 1 to 4 grams of omega-3 per day as needed for your desired effects.

Possible Side Effects

Fish oil can cause a fishy aftertaste and, rarely, stomach upset. This can be minimized by storing the fish oil in the freezer, removing a pill just prior to use.

Tips for Choosing a Brand of Fish Oil

Fishy aftertaste is more common with poor-quality fish oil that has already turned rancid. To check this out yourself, break open a fish oil capsule; it should have just the faintest fish odor. If it smells more like a garbage can, find another brand. Also, be sure to check the label for a statement that the oil has been tested for heavy metals; most popular brands are thoroughly tested, making fish oil more reliably free of toxins than the fish you eat.

Possible Interactions

Fish oil is a mild blood thinner and could interact with the potent prescription blood thinner warfarin (Coumadin); don't take fish oil if you take Coumadin.

Fish Oil and Heart Disease: Consider the Evidence

- Fish oil may help lower the risk of a heart attack. The Cardiovascular Health Study found that people with higher levels of omega-3 fatty acids had a lower risk of fatal heart attack.
- Eating fish helps reduce death rate in men recovering from heart attacks. A study of two thousand men recovering from heart attacks found that those eating fatty fish two or three times per week had a 29 percent reduction in their death rate over a two-year period, compared with individuals who did not eat fish.
- Fish oil helps lower triglyceride levels. In a four-week study, forty-seven healthy men taking 4 grams of fish oil daily (an amount corresponding to one to two weekly servings of fatty fish) saw a 30 percent decline in their plasma triglyceride levels.

NIACIN

Niacin is known as vitamin B_3 and nicotinic acid. Avoid nicotinamide or niacinamide, which have no cholesterol-lowering properties.

Comparing Niacin and Prescription Medications

The most effective agents known to lower LDL are statins, but niacin also has LDL-lowering properties. In addition, it raises HDL more than fibrates, a prescription drug used to lower triglycerides. See chapter 11 for a discussion of prescription medications.

How It Works

Niacin slows the production of harmful fats by the liver. It helps raise HDL and lower LDL, Lp(a), and triglyceride levels.

Using Niacin

Doses from 500 to 2,000 milligrams are used to improve cholesterol levels. Over-the-counter niacin is available in 100-, 250-, and 500-milligram tablets. An intermediate acting form of niacin, Niaspan (Kos Pharmaceuticals), is available only by prescription. Prescription niacin is no more effective than the over-the-counter form, though it does have the advantage of greater certainty of dosing—the content of supplements is not regulated.

Side Effects

Niacin, whether purchased over the counter or by prescription, has the potential to cause side effects including liver and muscle irritation, acid indigestion, and flaring of gout. It can also raise your blood sugar (glucose) level, although the effect, if any, is generally small. If you are a diabetic or pre-diabetic, sugar levels should be checked. For all of these reasons, anyone taking niacin supplements in any form should do so only under supervision of a physician.

A Word About a Common Niacin Problem—Flushing

The most common side effect of niacin is flushing. Flushing symptoms include facial blushing resembling a sunburn, as well as warmth and tingling of the skin. Flushing is an unpleasant nuisance, but it is not a risk to your health and causes no harm. This reaction is caused by niacin temporarily enlarging the small blood vessels under the skin. Flushing begins anywhere from thirty minutes to two hours after taking niacin and generally lasts less than an hour. If you experience this problem at first, don't give up—flushing generally becomes less intense the second, third, and fourth time you take niacin, and it often completely resolves within the first week. For some people, however, flushing does not improve appreciably over time. For these individuals, I often try to switch to a different brand. If flushing persists nevertheless, I generally discontinue niacin.

You can reduce the chance of flushing if you take niacin with food (usually in the evening), avoid alcohol or spicy food within two hours of taking niacin, and take aspirin (81 to 325 milligrams) with niacin (or up to one hour prior). If you forget to take aspirin before the niacin and you begin to flush, it is too late—aspirin works only before an episode.

Avoid "no-flush" or "flush-free" niacin. Because flushing is the biggest obstacle to taking niacin, some companies have produced an alternative form with promises that it avoids flushing. These preparations contain a bound-up type of niacin that many people cannot convert to the more active form. The result is often less flushing but, unfortunately, less benefit as well.

Niacin and Heart Disease: Consider the Evidence

- Niacin helps raise HDL, as well as lower LDL, Lp(a), and triglyceride levels. A multicenter, ninety-six-week study of five hundred men with elevated cholesterol found that niacin at doses between 1,000 and 2,000 milligrams lowered LDL cholesterol by 18 percent, increased HDL cholesterol by 29 percent, lowered triglycerides by 24 percent, and reduced Lp(a) by 36 percent.
- Niacin raises HDL cholesterol more effectively than the prescription cholesterol drug gemfibrozil. A multicenter trial involving 173 patients found that those taking niacin (1,500 to 2,000 milligrams daily) experienced twofold greater increases in HDL than those taking gemfibrozil (600 milligrams twice daily). In the study, the niacin at higher doses raised HDL levels by 26 percent, compared with 13 percent in the gemfibrozil group.

RED YEAST RICE

Red yeast rice is my agent of choice for those who need LDL treatment beyond lifestyle measures but cannot tolerate or wish to avoid prescription statins. It's also known as *Monascus purpureus.*

Comparing Red Yeast Rice and Prescription Medications

Prescription statins are the most potent LDL-lowering agents available. Red yeast rice, however, is the most potent over-the-counter product for lowering LDL cholesterol.

How It Works

Red yeast rice is the product of a yeast (*Monascus purpureus*) that when grown on rice under controlled conditions, produces a family of compounds known as monacolins. One of these is monacolin K, also known as lovastatin—the same statin sold by prescription under the brand name Mevacor. Red yeast rice is, therefore, an over-the-counter supplement that contains a naturally occurring type of statin that blocks the production of cholesterol by the liver. It also contains plant sterols that have additional cholesterol-lowering properties.

Red yeast rice may be a good alternative to statins for people with mild cholesterol elevation—less than 25 percent above their goal. It is an excellent option for patients who are opposed to taking a prescription statin or who have had side effects with several prescription products. I have many patients who are unable to tolerate prescription statins due to severe muscle pain but have been able to take red yeast rice without any adverse effects.

In order to maximize the cholesterol-lowering effect, I often add red yeast rice to either over-the-counter plant stanols/sterols (discussed below) or prescription Zetia (discussed in chapter 11). Using these combinations, I have been able to achieve LDL lowering of 30 to 55 percent.

Using Red Yeast Rice

The starting dose is 600 milligrams taken twice a day; the maximum dose is 1,200 milligrams taken twice a day.

Possible Side Effects

Red yeast rice, like other statins, can cause muscle and liver irritation, although less frequently than with prescription statins in my experience. Red yeast rice, like prescription statins, can lower CoQ10 levels (see below).

Possible Interactions

Avoid using red yeast rice with prescription statins. The two work via identical mechanisms, and the combination could increase the risk of side effects. When used with over-the-counter niacin or several other prescription medications (including some antibiotics), the risk of liver and muscle irritation increases. I strongly recommend that red yeast rice be taken only under a doctor's supervision.

Red Yeast Rice and Heart Disease: Consider the Evidence

• Taking red yeast rice can significantly lower LDL cholesterol and triglycerides. A double-blind, placebo-controlled, twelve-week study of eighty-three healthy subjects with high cholesterol found that participants who took 2.4 grams of red yeast rice daily experienced a 23 percent drop in their LDL cholesterol, compared with those who received a placebo.

STANOLS/STEROLS

Stanols are also known as sitostanol, and plant stanol; sterols are sometimes called sitosterol, phytosterol, and plant sterols.

Comparing Stanols/Sterols and Prescription Medications

Zetia and WelChol are prescription medications that work in the digestive tract to lower LDL cholesterol, as do stanols and sterols. In my experience, stanols and sterols are mildly less potent than these prescription medications.

How They Work

Mammalian cells contain chole*sterol*; plant cells contain phyto-*sterol*. Plant sterols help lower cholesterol because they bind up the docking stations in the digestive tract usually reserved for cholesterol. The result is that less cholesterol gets absorbed into the bloodstream, and cholesterol levels plummet. Sterols can be slightly chemically altered to form stanols, a form that dissolves more easily than sterols. Both sterols and stanols are effective at lowering cholesterol.

Using Stanols/Sterols

I frequently use stanols and sterols in my practice. For some patients, the use of stanols and sterols alone is adequate to achieve desired cholesterol levels. For people with more difficult problems, I add stanols and sterols to other treatments as boosters. I prefer stanols and sterols in pill form; these are easy to take and more convenient for most people. With 2 grams of stanols/sterols per day, you can expect a 10 to 20 percent reduction in LDL levels.

In addition, stanols and sterols are available in certain margarines, including Take Control and Benecol. My experience is that few people wish to consume the 2 to 4 tablespoons of margarine daily needed to yield that much active ingredient.

Another limitation of using these special margarines for therapy is that it can be difficult for people who eat out or travel often.

Possible Side Effects

Stanols/sterols are extremely well tolerated. Very rare side effects include indigestion, gas, diarrhea, or constipation.

Possible Interactions

Sterols may reduce absorption of fat-soluble nutrients, including vitamn E and beta-carotene.

Stanols/Sterols and Heart Disease: Consider the Evidence

- Stanols reduce LDL and total cholesterol, but have little effect on HDL. A one-year double-blind study of 153 people with mildly elevated cholesterol found that people consuming margarine containing sitostanol ester had a mean 10.2 percent reduction in total cholesterol, compared with an increase of 0.1 percent in the control group. The reduction in LDL cholesterol was 14.1 percent in the stanol group and 1.1 percent in the control group. HDL cholesterol and triglyceride levels were unchanged.
- Sterols also reduce LDL and total cholesterol, but have little effect on HDL. A sixteen-week double-blind study of sixty-two people with high cholesterol found that those consuming margarine enriched with plant sterols experienced a reduction in LDL cholesterol of 10 to 15

percent compared with those in the control group; HDL and triglyceride levels were unchanged.

COENZYME Q10

Coenzyme Q10 is also known as ubiquinol and ubiquinone. It does not have a prescription drug equivalent.

How It Works

Coenzyme Q10 is a vitaminlike compound present in virtually all cells; it's found in especially high concentrations in the heart. Its primary functions include activity as an antioxidant and as a helper in many metabolic pathways, particularly in the production of the body's prime energy currency, adenosine triphosphate (ATP). The body produces coenzyme Q10 naturally in addition to obtaining some from a wide variety of foods. Levels are highest during the first twenty years of life and decline with age. The use of statin drugs significantly reduces coenzyme Q10 levels (see chapter 11). For this reason, I recommend that all my patients taking prescription statins or red yeast rice also consider taking coenzyme Q10 supplements. There is some evidence that such supplementation may prevent the muscle irritation sometimes experienced with statin medication. Other researched uses include treatment of hypertension and congestive heart failure.

Using Coenzyme Q10

Take 100 milligrams daily when using statins; take 200 to 300 milligrams daily for hypertension and congestive heart failure.

Possible Interactions

Coenzyme Q10 may reduce the blood-thinning effect of warfarin (Coumadin); do not take CoQ10 if you take warfarin.

Coenzyme Q10 and Heart Disease: Consider the Evidence

- Coenzyme Q10 helps improve symptoms of congestive heart failure. A study of more than six hundred people with congestive heart failure found that those who took coenzyme Q10 experienced fewer hospitalizations than the control group, and they had half the rate of serious complications.
- Coenzyme Q10 helps lower blood pressure. A study of more than one hundred patients with hypertension found that those taking coenzyme Q10 experienced a gradual decrease in their blood pressure; more than half the study participants no longer needed between one and three medications for hypertension within four months of taking CoQ10. (The average dose in the study was 225 milligrams per day.)
- Coenzyme Q10 helps decrease the risk of cardiac events in people who have had recent heart attacks. In a randomized, double-blind study, 141 people who had had heart attacks were divided into two groups. The first received 120 milligrams of coenzyme Q10 daily, while the second received a placebo. After one year, the number of cardiac problems—including heart attacks—was significantly lower in the group taking CoQ10.

L-CARNITINE

Comparing Carnitine and Prescription Medications

L-carnitine lowers Lp(a), although much less effectively than niacin (prescription or over the counter). In my prevention practice, I use L-carnitine to help lower Lp(a) in patients for whom niacin is inadequate or cannot be used because of side effects.

How It Works

L-carnitine is found throughout the body. It plays a key role in energy production in the mitochondria, our body's natural power plants.

Using Carnitine

Take 1 gram of L-carnitine twice a day.

Possible Side Effects

On rare occasions, L-carnitine can cause nausea and diarrhea.

Possible Interactions

L-carnitine may increase the potency of the blood-thinning medicine warfarin (Coumadin).

Check the Label

Be sure to take L-carnitine rather than D-carnitine, a form that can interfere with the effectiveness of L-carnitine.

L-Carnitine and Heart Disease: Consider the Evidence

- L-carnitine lowers Lp(a) levels in the blood. A study of thirty-six people with elevated Lp(a) levels found that those who received 2 grams of L-carnitine daily had an 8 percent reduction in Lp(a) levels. The most dramatic reductions occurred in people with the highest readings.

VITAMIN D

Vitamin D is also known as cholecalciferol and ergocalciferol. It does not have a prescription medication equivalent.

How It Works

Vitamin D is a fat-soluble vitamin that regulates calcium and phosphorus levels. Although it does not alter cholesterol levels appreciably, there is mounting evidence that it has an impact on the heart in other important ways. The connection between vitamin D and heart health is supported by the observation that heart attacks are much more frequent in the winter and in higher latitudes, situations where vitamin D levels are low due to less exposure to sunlight. The risk of heart attacks is twice as high for those with low vitamin D levels in the blood (below 34 ng/mL), compared with those above this level. Optimal levels are above 40 ng/mL. Vitamin D may also play a role in determining blood pressure; treatment with ultraviolet light and oral supplementation with vitamin D have been shown to have a significant impact on reducing high blood pressure.

Using Vitamin D

Vitamin D is obtained from three sources: skin production in response to sunlight, dietary consumption, and supplements. Foods rich in vitamin D include salmon, fortified milk, and sardines. The vitamin D manufactured in the skin and consumed in the diet is vitamin D_3 (cholecalciferol)—the preferred form. An alternative form, ergocalciferol or vitamin D_2, is not as efficient as D_3 and should generally not be used.

Vitamin D supplements may be considered for those with documented low blood levels (see above), people with limited sun exposure, and those living in northern latitudes.

Vitamin D supplements should be taken in the form of cholecalciferol (D_3) at a typical dose of 1,000 International Units (IU) daily.

Possible Side Effects

Vitamin D in daily doses of 1,000 IU or less tends to be well tolerated without side effects.

Possible Interactions

Vitamin D may cause a problem when taken with thiazide diuretics—combined use can lead to a buildup of calcium in the blood.

Vitamin D and Heart Disease: Consider the Evidence

- Vitamin D deficiency has been linked to increased risk of heart attack. A group of 179 patients who had suffered heart attacks were compared with a comparable control group that had not experienced cardiac events. Researchers found those who had heart attacks had significantly lower blood levels of vitamin D than the people in the control group.

- Vitamin D along with calcium helps lower systolic blood pressure. An eight-week study involving 148 women found that those who received 1,200 milligrams of calcium plus 800 IU of vitamin D experienced a decrease in systolic blood pressure of 9.3 percent and a decrease in heart rate of 5.4 percent.

SHOULD YOU TAKE DAILY ASPIRIN?

While most patients add aspirin to their healthy heart regimens at the recommendation of their doctors, aspirin is available over the counter, so I have included it in the discussion of other supplements. Dozens of clinical trials support the use of aspirin to prevent heart attack and stroke. Aspirin is most beneficial for prevention of heart disease and stroke in those forty or older who have other significant vascular risk factors as described earlier in this book.

Data on aspirin show it truly to be a wonder drug, with a reduction in the risk of heart disease and stroke of up to 30 percent in some studies. Those without significant risk factors for vascular disease are less likely to benefit.

There is no clear consensus regarding the optimal dose of aspirin to prevent heart disease or stroke. For those without a history of heart attack or stroke, a dose of aspirin between 81 milligrams (referred to as a "baby aspirin") and 162 milligrams per day is likely sufficient. Those with a history of heart disease or stroke are most commonly treated with a dose between 162 and 325 milligrams per day.

While supplements play an essential role in heart health, they cannot make up for a poor diet. As discussed in the following chapter, supplements and diet work together to nourish the body and maintain a healthy heart.

TAKE THIS TO HEART

Which supplements do you need? I recommend:

- Fish oil (1 to 4 grams daily) to everyone. Fish oil can lower triglycerides 25 to 40 percent, reduce inflammation, and convert small, dense LDL into the more favorable large, fluffy type.
- Niacin (500 to 2,000 milligrams daily) to those with low HDL, high LDL, high Lp(a), high triglycerides, and small, dense LDL. It's used to raise HDL and lower LDL and Lp(a) by 15 to 30 percent. It can also convert small, dense LDL into the more favorable large, fluffy form.
- Red yeast rice (600 to 1,200 milligrams twice a day with food) to those with high LDL who cannot tolerate or wish to avoid prescription statins. It can lower LDL cholesterol by about 25 percent.
- Stanols and sterols (2 grams daily) to those with high LDL. Those can lower LDL 10 to 20 percent.

- Coenzyme Q10 (100 to 300 milligrams daily) to those on statins, to replace depleted coenzyme Q10 and possibly lower blood pressure and improve symptoms of heart failure.
- L-carnitine (1 gram twice a day) to those with high Lp(a), to lower Lp(a) level by 8 percent.
- Vitamin D (1,000 IU taken in the form of vitamin D_3 or cholecalciferol) to those living in conditions of low sun exposure or with documented low blood levels of vitamin D. This supplement can lower the risk of heart disease.

———— ◆◆ ————

Chapter 7

Eat Right:
Lowering Cholesterol with Diet

We often drive our bodies like high-performance sports cars, while fueling them like junkers. Our bodies can perform reasonably well for years on low-quality fuel, but resiliency declines over time. All too often, that means heart disease somewhere down the road.

This chapter will focus on some very simple, yet powerful, concepts that form the foundation of a healthy heart diet. One important bonus of heart-healthy eating: It is likely that you will also lose weight. If you make the right food choices (most of the time), your body will slim down naturally, without counting calories or turning to a strict weight-loss plan. Rather than approaching food with the goal of losing weight, approach food with a goal of eating right—*and the weight loss will take care of itself.*

When I discuss dietary change with my patients, I typically don't sit down with them and set a weight goal. Instead, I encourage them to eat more of certain healthy foods and less of other harmful foods, as described in this chapter. If you follow the four key principles outlined here, you will improve your cholesterol profile and lose excess weight:

- **Eat the right fats.** Choose healthy monounsaturated fats and omega-3s, reduce saturated fats, and eliminate trans fats.
- **Choose whole foods.** The closer to nature, the better. Avoid preservatives and additives.
- **Emphasize carbohydrates with a low gylcemic load rating.** Avoid foods that raise blood sugar levels quickly.
- **Limit your intake of high-fructose corn syrup.** This refined sugar is added to many processed foods but creates unique health problems.

Many of these core principles also provide the cornerstones of an anti-inflammatory diet, an approach to eating popularized by Dr. Andrew Weil and described in his 2005 book *Healthy Aging.* The healthy foods included in this diet help reduce levels of inflammation and lower the risk of plaque formation and heart disease (as described in chapter 2).

If you follow these simple guidelines, which I explain in detail below, you probably will see measurable changes in your cholesterol numbers and weight within about two months. Of course, the greater the magnitude of change in your diet, the greater the magnitude of change you'll see in your cholesterol numbers. Someone shifting from a diet of bacon cheeseburgers and fries to spinach salads and broiled salmon is more likely to notice a significant drop in cholesterol than someone who just needed to make a few minor adjustments to what was essentially a fairly well-balanced diet.

While making wise diet choices benefits everyone, some people tend to be more responsive to dietary changes than others. You may know someone with a desirable cholesterol profile and less-than-admirable eating habits, and someone else who follows a strict diet but still struggles with elevated cholesterol scores that don't want to budge. This may seem unfair, but to some degree your body's response to dietary changes is influenced by your genes. Even without significant changes in your cholesterol levels, you will still be nourishing your body with foods that provide other benefits, including possibly helping to prevent heart disease, cancer, and diabetes, among other problems.

RULE 1: EAT THE RIGHT FATS

Fats, although often vilified, are essential to human health; they are needed for growth, hormone production, and other essential body processes. They also carry and store fat-soluble vitamins (vitamins A, D, E, and K). And of course, fats make food more palatable by adding flavor, aroma, and texture.

Not all fats are created equal. Dietary fats consist of combinations of three types: saturated, polyunsaturated, and monounsaturated, as well as a mostly human-made version known as trans fat. Rather than working to reduce all fats in your diet, I suggest that you learn which fats are healthy and which should be minimized or avoided.

Saturated Fat: Limit as Much as Possible

Saturated fat is among the most potent fuels to raise bad LDL cholesterol levels and increase the risk of heart disease. Foods high in saturated fat include butter, cheese, egg yolk (but not white), whole milk, red meat, skin on poultry, and palm oil.

Many of my patients are cheese lovers; I can relate to this

addiction myself. Most people are surprised to learn that certain types of cheese have ounce for ounce twice as much saturated fat as red meat. My advice is to choose low-fat brands of cheese, and limit the overall amount. For example, you might avoid extra slices of cheese on sandwiches and use low-fat versions whenever possible. Even pizza shops often offer this as an option these days, and my experience is that the taste is indistinguishable from full-fat cheese.

Another concern is adequate protein intake. Many of us take in most of our protein from foods containing high levels of saturated fat, including red meat and full-fat dairy. A diet low in saturated fat still leaves plenty of room for protein intake, however, including white meat, chicken without skin, fish, small portions of lean beef, no-fat dairy, beans, tofu, and nuts.

Read nutritional labels and compare the content of saturated fat among brands; use low saturated fat content as one of the criteria in making your food choices.

CONFUSION ABOUT CHOLESTEROL IN FOOD

Food ads about cholesterol can often be misleading. Cholesterol is found only in animal products. Some products are marketed as "no cholesterol" as a special lure, despite the fact that they never contain an animal product and, therefore, would not be expected to have cholesterol in the first place. So a claim for a special "no-cholesterol peanut butter" is nonsense, because peanut butter—not being an animal product—never contains cholesterol.

Also, don't assume that a product labeled "no cholesterol and fat-free" is necessarily heart-healthy. Many such foods are loaded with sugar, trading off one health problem for another. Read labels carefully and completely.

Monounsaturated Fats: A Heart-Healthy Choice

Monounsaturated fats have been shown to lower the level of bad LDL cholesterol and raise good HDL cholesterol levels when they replace saturated fats in the diet. Monounsaturated fats are the key oils in the healthy Mediterranean diet, which derives most of its fat calories from olive oil and olives. Foods high in monounsaturated fats include olive oil, olives, canola oil, avocados, and nuts.

Polyunsaturated Fats (Especially Omega-3): A Heart-Healthy Choice

Polyunsatured fats come in two forms: omega-3 and omega-6. Both are necessary for good health. The typical American, however, consumes far too much omega-6 and too little omega-3 (see below). Here are some other important facts:

- Omega-3 fatty acids lower LDL cholesterol.
- Diets higher in polyunsaturated and monounsaturated fats are linked to lower risk of heart disease.
- Diets high in omega-3 fatty acids lower triglycerides and reduce the risk of cardiovascular disease. Studies have found that people who consume two or more servings of fish (which is high in omega-3s) per week have a 30 percent decrease in risk of cardiovascular disease.

OMEGA-3 FATTY ACIDS IN FISH

Following is the omega-3 fatty acid content of a 3.5-ounce serving of various fish:

Mackerel	2.6 grams
Trout, lake	2.0
Herring	1.7
Tuna, bluefin	1.6
Salmon	1.5
Sardines, canned	1.5
Sturgeon, Atlantic	1.5
Tuna, albacore	1.5
Bass, striped	0.8
Trout, rainbow	0.6
Bass, freshwater	0.3
Snapper, red	0.2
Swordfish	0.2

In order to limit the risk of mercury toxicity from fish, my advice is to choose wild fish over farm-raised varieties (unless they are organic), and to limit intake of those larger fish, such as tuna and swordfish, that tend to collect more toxins.

Understanding Omega-3s and Omega-6s

Our distant hunter-gatherer ancestors ate lots of fish, green plants, and berries. This diet included plenty of omega-3 and omega-6 fatty acids, probably in roughly equal amounts. Our modern diet, on the other hand, is loaded with processed foods and vegetable oils, which tip the ratio of omega-6s to omega-3s to as high as 20:1—or twenty times more omega-6s than omega-3s. This is a problem because omega-6 fatty acids boost the level of inflammation in the body, while omega-3s are decidedly anti-inflammatory.

Bottom line: Eat more omega-3 and fewer omega-6 fatty acids.

- **Sources of omega-3 fatty acids** include fish, fish oil, ground flaxseeds and flaxseed oil, soy products, nuts, dark green leafy vegetables, and "omega-3 enhanced" eggs.
- **Sources of omega-6 fatty acids** include corn, safflower, cottonseed, sesame, and sunflower oils, as well as margarine, traditional eggs (as opposed to "omega-3 enhanced"), and baked goods.

FISH OIL OR FLAX?

Many people want to supplement the omega-3 content of their diet but are confused about which is better: flax or fish oil? Fish oil is the winner, because it contains the form of oil most easily used by your body. Flax oil, on the other hand, requires conversion in the body to the more usable form. Many people have a limited capacity to make this chemical conversion and so, for them, flax is not an efficient source of omega-3. For this reason, my general preference is fish oil over flax. Better yet, use fish oil supplements and, in addition, sprinkle some freshly ground flaxseeds on your yogurt or cereal for added benefit.

Trans Fats: Avoid Completely

These are the most dangerous of all fats; they are highly efficient at increasing your cholesterol level and promoting the plaque that causes heart disease and stroke. Food manufacturers create trans fats by bubbling hydrogen through vegetable oil in a process known as hydrogenation. Trans fats are added to foods to increase their shelf life (while shortening yours). There is no safe level of trans fats: The best diet has a trans fat intake of zero. Other facts you should know about trans fats:

- Trans fats increase CRP levels.
- Trans fats increase lipoprotein (a) levels.
- Trans fats increase triglyceride levels.
- Trans fats are linked to an increased risk of cardiovascular disease.

Examples of trans fats include partially hydrogenated oils (check product labels), traditional margarine (especially stick margarine), vegetable shortening, fried foods, commercially prepared baked goods, doughnuts, potato chips, and fast foods.

Types of Fat in Common Oils

The heart-healthy oils are listed in all capital letters.

Oil	Percent Saturated Fat	Percent Monounsaturated Fat	Percent Polyunsaturated Fat	Percent Trans Fat
AVOCADO	11	71	14	4
Butter	60	30	5	5

CANOLA	**6**	**62**	**31**	**1**
Corn	13	25	62	0
Lard	41	47	12	0
OLIVE	**14**	**77**	**9**	**0**
Palm	51	39	10	0
Peanut	13	49	33	5
SAFFLOWER	**9**	**12**	**78**	**1**
Sunflower	10	20	66	4

Change Your Diet Today: Eat Healthier Fats

- Do eat cold-water fish twice a week.
- Do opt for olive oil rather than butter on bread or creamy dressings on salad.
- Do eat nuts for snacks in place of cookies or chips.
- Do choose omega-3 enhanced eggs rather than conventional eggs.
- Do drink skim milk rather than 2 percent.
- Do remove the skin from chicken and other poultry.

RULE 2: CHOOSE WHOLE FOODS

As a general rule, if a food comes in a package, it's not your best bet. The less a food is processed, the healthier it is for you—because of both what the food contains (more nutrients) and what it does not (additives and preservatives). Healthy choices do exist in some packaged foods (such as whole-grain breads or dried fruits), but these foods should have as few added ingredients as possible.

Choose Whole Grains

Most grains in a typical American diet are artificially refined. Whole grains contain the outer shell (or bran) as well as the germ, or potential seedling; they are high in fiber, vitamins, complex carbohydrates, and minerals. Refined grains have been stripped of much of their fiber, essential fatty acids, and phytochemicals (chemical nutrients found in plants); some manufacturers try to make up for this deficit by enriching the foods with some vitamins and minerals. Bread should be labeled "100 percent whole wheat" rather than just "wheat" to ensure you are choosing a whole-grain product.

Eat Fruits and Vegetables

The benefits of eating fruits and vegetables are widely known. Unlike processed foods, fresh fruits and vegetables are packed with nutrients and relatively low in calories. Their phytochemicals and antioxidants are our best natural protection against heart disease (as well as cancer). Nature has an amazing system for keeping us healthy: Fruit and vegetables come color-coded! Each color contains a unique health-promoting nutrient.

In a study of eighty-four thousand women and forty-two thousand men, those who ate the most fruits and vegetables, particularly green leafy vegetables and vitamin-C-rich fruits and vegetables, experienced the lowest risk of cardiovascular disease. (Increased consumption of potatoes was not associated with benefits.)

Eat Plenty of Fiber

A diet high in whole foods will naturally be high in fiber. While not a nutrient, dietary fiber is a vital part of a well-balanced diet. It's made of complex carbohydrates, the substances that give structure and shape to plants. There are two types of fiber—soluble and insoluble—both of which are found in fruits, vegetables, legumes, and whole grains.

- **Soluble fiber** dissolves during digestion, forming a gel-like material that traps cholesterol in the digestive tract where it can be eliminated. Foods high in soluble fiber include oats, kidney beans, citrus fruits, apples, and potatoes.
- **Insoluble fiber,** as the name implies, does not dissolve in water as it moves through the digestive system. This type of fiber provides the stools with the bulk required to absorb body waste; it also helps the intestines work smoothly and speeds the movement of stools through the intestines. Wheat bran and whole grains, as well as the skins of many fruits and vegetables, are rich sources of this type of fiber.

Current guidelines recommend that the average adult consume at least 25 grams of fiber daily by eating a diet rich in fruits, vegetables, and whole grains. Most Americans eat less than half the fiber they need. In general, the less processed or refined a food is, the more fiber it contains.

A 1996 study published in the *Journal of the American Medical Association* found that men who ate more than 25 grams of fiber per day had a 36 percent lower risk of developing heart disease than those who consumed less than 15 grams. The study found that every 10 grams of fiber added to the diet lowered the risk of heart attack by 19 percent.

Soluble fiber is a powerful natural option to lower your cholesterol. You can reduce LDL cholesterol by up to 5 percent by adding 5 grams per day of soluble fiber to your diet (one apple, one orange, and one carrot a day).

How Much Fiber Are You Eating?

	Serving Size:	Total Fiber (g)	Soluble Fiber (g)
Grains			
Bran, wheat, dry	½ cup	6	Trace (less than 1 g)
Spaghetti (whole wheat)	1 cup	4	1
Rice, brown, cooked	½ cup	2	Trace
Spaghetti	1 cup	2	1
Whole wheat bread	1 slice	2	Trace
White bread	1 slice	1	Trace
Legumes			
Lima beans	½ cup	7	3
Beans, baked	½ cup	6	3
Kidney beans	½ cup	6	3
Green peas, cooked	½ cup	4	1
Peanuts, dry-roasted	¼ cup	3	1
Fruits			
Pear, fresh	1 large	5	3
Apple, fresh	1 large	4	1
Plum, fresh	5 small	4	2
Banana, fresh	1 medium	3	1

Fruits (*continued*)

Orange, fresh	1 medium	3	1
Peach, fresh	1 medium	2	1
Raisins	¼ cup	2	Trace

Vegetables

Parsnips, cooked	½ cup	4	2
Carrots, cooked	½ cup	3	1
Potato, baked (with skin)	1 medium	3	1
Squash, winter, cooked	½ cup	3	2
Corn, cooked	½ cup	2	Trace
Broccoli, cooked	½ cup	1	1

Cereals

Fiber One	½ cup	14	1
All-Bran	⅔ cup	13	1
100% Bran	½ cup	12	1
Raisin bran	¾ cup	6	1
Oatmeal	1 cup	4	2
Cheerios	1¼ cups	4	1
Wheaties	1 cup	2	1
Special K	1⅓ cups	1	Trace

Source: Minnesota Nutrient Data Base, Tufts University School of Medicine, Boston

Eat High-Folate Foods

Foods high in folate and other B vitamins help lower homo-cysteine levels and reduce the risk of cardiovascular disease. Food rich in folate acid include green leafy vegetables, asparagus, oranges, strawberries, melons, and whole wheat products.

Eat Soy-Based Foods

Soy foods—soybeans, tofu, miso, soy milk, soy protein, and textured vegetable protein—can help lower cholesterol. In fact, the US Food and Drug Administration has approved the health claim that consuming 25 grams of soy protein daily helps reduce the risk of heart disease, when taken with a low-fat diet.

Soy owes much of its heart-healthy reputation to a family of active ingredients called isoflavones. This group of compounds is responsible for lowering LDL cholesterol and reducing the risk of heart disease. Soybeans are a good source of vitamins, minerals, protein, and unsaturated fat. Soy protein also helps to meet the dietary demands for protein and can replace protein sources high in saturated fat.

Change Your Diet: Eat Whole Foods

- Do eat whole wheat cereals, pastas, breads, and baked goods.
- Do snack on fresh vegetables and fruit. Aim for a minimum of three servings of each per day (five each is optimal, but if adding fruit and vegetables to your diet is a new idea for you, aiming for three each to begin with is a good start). How can you eat three of each quickly? Well, a large salad for lunch counts as two vegetable servings; adding a side vegetable to dinner gives you three for the day. With fruits, try adding berries to your breakfast, having a banana for a midmorning snack, and eating an apple midafternoon or with dinner.
- Do add as many different colors of fruits and vegetables

in your daily diet as possible: Each color contains a different healthy nutrient.

- Do opt for brown rice instead of white.
- Do add wheat germ to cereal or yogurt.
- Do eat skins on potatoes, apples, and other fruits and vegetables with edible skins.

RULE 3: EMPHASIZE CARBOHYDRATES WITH A LOW GLYCEMIC LOAD RATING

Maintaining a normal blood sugar level is essential to heart health. (Remember, diabetes and pre-diabetes both put you at increased risk of heart attack.) Carbohydrates are the elements of food that most strongly influence the sugar level. Carbohydrates can be further divided into *simple* (sugars, including fructose, glucose, and sucrose) and *complex* (long chains of sugars arranged to form starches and fiber). Simple carbohydrates have an immediate and dramatic impact on raising blood sugar levels, while complex carbohydrates are absorbed more slowly and do not tend to raise sugar levels as high.

You can use a food's glycemic index and glycemic load to measure its effect on blood sugar levels and to help you make wise food choices. The *glycemic index* is a measurement of how quickly a food is converted into sugar in the body. Foods with lower glycemic index values are preferred because they do not tend to boost sugar levels as much as high-glycemic foods. This issue is especially important for people who have a problem handling sugar, including those with pre-diabetes (fasting blood sugar levels of 100 to 125 mg/dL) as well as those with established diabetes (fasting sugar of more than 125 mg/dL).

In order to make the best estimate of how much a given food is likely to increase your sugar level, you must consider both the glycemic index of the food and the amount of carbohydrate contained in a typical serving. Fortunately, this grand total figure is readily available in a number known as the *glycemic load.*

In essence, the glycemic load takes into account both the quality and the quantity of carbohydrate. Take, for example, watermelon, a food with a high glycemic index but a fairly low glycemic load (see the chart on page 108). This difference reflects the fact that a 100-gram serving has only 6 grams of available carbohydrate per serving; fiber is a carbohydrate that is not absorbed by the body so it does not contribute to the glycemic load.

High-glycemic carbohydrates head straight for the liver, where they are broken down into glucose or sugar. The pancreas then kicks into gear, producing insulin to move the sugar into the cells. The sugar can be used for energy (causing the so-called sugar rush). Both the liver and the muscles store as much glucose as they can (in the form of glycogen), but eventually, the rest of the calories get tucked away as fat.

Understanding the glycemic load helps to explain why so many weight-loss diets fail. Many dieters restrict their overall calories and fat consumption, but continue to eat high-glycemic foods. These foods—some eaten in the guise of "healthy low-fat foods"—lead to sugar spikes in the blood, and eventual conversion into fat.

In addition, simple carbohydrates—which tend to be high on the glycemic index—are converted into triglycerides. Triglycerides and HDL have a teeter-totter relationship: When triglycerides are high, HDL plummets. Therefore, high-glycemic foods contribute to heart disease by increasing triglyceride levels and decreasing the level of healthy HDL. The strong link between a high-glycemic diet and cardiovascular risk was shown in a ten-year study of more than seventy-five thousand women; the risk of heart disease was greatest in those who were overweight and ate high-glycemic foods.

In addition, eating a high-glycemic diet appears to fire up the body's inflammatory response, as reflected in higher levels of C-reactive protein. A study of 244 healthy, middle-aged women found a strong association between dietary glycemic load and CRP levels, especially among overweight women.

In order to improve your cholesterol profile, cool your body's inflammatory reaction, and lose weight, you need to minimize your intake of high-glycemic foods. Some of the figures may surprise you, so take a few minutes to study the glycemic load chart that follows. It is impossible to guess how much certain foods raise sugar levels by how sweet they taste. For example, most people would assume that a candy bar has a much higher glycemic load than a white bagel but, in fact, the two are nearly identical in their impact on sugar levels.

The Glycemic Load of Common Foods

The following chart rates common carbohydrates based on their glycemic load. Low-glycemic foods tend not to raise blood sugar levels as dramatically as high-glycemic foods. For additional data on the glycemic load of common foods, refer to a book from your local library, such as *The New Glucose Revolution Shopper's Guide to GI Values* 2006 by Dr. Jennie Brand-Miller and Kaye Foster-Powell (Marlow, 2006).

Food	Serving Size	Glycemic Load
Fruit		
Cherries	4.2 oz.	3
Grapefruit	4.2 oz.	3
Apples	4.2 oz.	6
Oranges	4.2 oz.	5
Peaches	4.2 oz.	5
Grapes	4.2 oz.	8
Orange juice	8.4 oz.	13
Pears	4.2 oz.	4
Bananas	4.2 oz.	12
Raisins	2.1 oz.	28
Cantaloupe	4.2 oz.	4
Pineapple	4.2 oz.	7
Watermelon	4.2 oz.	4
Starchy Vegetables		
Sweet potatoes	5.3 oz.	17
Yams	5.3 oz.	13
Beets	2.8 oz.	5
Couscous	5.3 oz.	23
White potatoes	5.3 oz.	18
French fries	5.3 oz.	22
Instant potatoes	5.3 oz.	17
Carrots	2.8 oz.	3
Parsnips	2.8 oz.	12

Dairy Products

Skim milk	8.8 oz.	4
Whole milk	8.8 oz.	3
Ice cream	1.8 oz.	8
Yogurt, no sugar	7 oz.	3

Legumes

Soybeans	5.3 oz.	1
Lentils	5.3 oz.	5
Black-eyed peas	5.3 oz.	13
Garbanzo beans	5.3 oz.	8
Baked beans	5.3 oz.	7
Frozen peas	5.3 oz.	2

Pasta, Corn, Rice, Bread

Spaghetti	3.2 oz.	9
Whole wheat pasta	3.2 oz.	8
Sweet corn	2.8 oz.	9
Blueberry muffin	2.0 oz.	17
Brown rice	5.3 oz.	18
White bread	1.1 oz.	10
Whole wheat bread	1.1 oz.	9
White rice	5.3 oz.	23
Bagel, white	2.5 oz.	25
Rice cake	0.9 oz.	17
Pretzel	1.1 oz.	16
Baguette	1.1 oz.	15

Breakfast Cereals

Oatmeal	1.1 oz.	2
All-Bran	1.1 oz.	6
Shredded wheat	1.1 oz.	15
Cornflakes	1.1 oz.	21

Miscellaneous

Peanuts	1.8 oz.	1
Tomato soup	8.8 oz.	6
Potato chips	1.8 oz.	11
Mars bar	2.1 oz.	26

Change Your Diet: Eat Low-Glycemic Foods

- Do become familiar with the glycemic load of your favorite foods. Remember, you can't necessarily predict which foods will have low or high glycemic loads; you need to do a bit of research. (One hour of reading will go a long way!)
- Do emphasize whole foods over processed products.
- Do minimize your intake of cookies, cake, white breads, white rice, potatoes, chips, and crackers.

RULE 4: LIMIT YOUR INTAKE OF HIGH-FRUCTOSE CORN SYRUP

High-fructose corn syrup is an artificially manipulated sweetener that became popular in the 1970s. It can be found in many processed foods containing added sweeteners, including soft drinks, breakfast cereals, canned fruits, jellies, flavored yogurts, baked goods, condiments, and prepared desserts. While simple sugars of any type should be kept to a minimum, this type of sweetener triggers a cascade of health problems all its own.

Consumption of high-fructose corn syrup increased by more than 1,000 percent between 1970 and 1990, mirroring the skyrocketing rates of obesity in America.

Why is high-fructose corn syrup a special problem? The body metabolizes fructose differently from other sugars. Normally, carbohydrates trigger the release of insulin, which, in turn, triggers the release of leptin, a hormone that signals fullness and satisfaction. Unlike other sugars, however, fructose does not stimulate insulin secretion in the pancreas or the release of leptin, so the body does not receive the message to stop eating. In other words, the sugary foods and soft drinks containing high-fructose corn syrup not only pack on pounds with empty calories, but also undermine the body's natural signals to regulate eating.

Metabolically, too, the body handles high-fructose corn syrup differently from other sugars; it is more readily metabolized into fat in the liver. It also raises triglyceride levels and is linked to high blood sugar levels as well as high blood pressure.

The traditional concept of being overweight relates to an imbalance of calories in and calories out. High-fructose corn syrup is an example of why this theory is incomplete. A given number of calories from high-fructose corn syrup present a more overwhelming metabolic challenge to the body than the same number of calories from another, natural source. Bottom line: Not all calories are created equal.

Choosing whole foods rather than processed foods will help limit consumption of high-fructose corn syrup. In addition, avoid sugared soft drinks and read product labels carefully.

Change Your Diet: Avoid High-Fructose Corn Syrup

- Do check the labels of food in your refrigerator and pantry; discard items that list high-fructose corn syrup.
- Do check labels on all food items you buy (including soft drinks, snacks, and condiments) and avoid purchasing those that list high-fructose corn syrup as a main ingredient.

WHAT TO CHOOSE WHEN EATING OUT OR ON THE ROAD

Many people can follow a healthy meal plan when eating at home but lose sight of their diet program when a menu is placed before them. The following tips can help you eat well when you eat out:

- Choose fish instead of poultry or red meat, but order it broiled or baked rather than fried.
- Choose a salad with vinaigrette rather than a cream-based dressing.
- If you want dessert, order sorbet or in-season berries.
- Avoid sauces or order them on the side to avoid drenching your food in high-calorie and high-fat toppings.

A HEART-HEALTHY MENU

Breakfast

- Orange juice, fortified with calcium.
- Main meal (one of the following): whole-grain cold

cereal (no added sugar) with low-fat soy or skim milk; low-fat yogurt sprinkled with wheat germ; hot oatmeal (not instant) with fresh fruit; "omega-3 enhanced" egg, white only; or whole wheat English muffin or toast with natural, no-sugar-added preserves.

- Fresh fruit.
- Green tea or coffee.

Lunch

- Main meal (one of the following): tuna salad with little dressing; turkey or chicken breast sandwich on whole wheat bread (no cheese); salad with vinaigrette dressing or a small amount of low-fat dressing (could include grilled chicken); or vegetarian chili.
- Fresh fruit.

Dinner

- Salad with vinaigrette or small amount of low-fat dressing.
- Main meal (one of the following): fish (not fried); chicken or turkey (no skin); or whole wheat pasta.
- Stir-fried or steamed vegetables.
- Fresh fruit.

Snacks

- Almonds or walnuts (one handful per day).
- Baby carrots or celery.
- Soy nuts.
- Fresh fruit.

TAKE THIS TO HEART

- Switch to heart-healthy fats: Eat more monounsaturated and omega-3 fatty acids; limit saturated fats; and avoid all trans fats.
- Eat whole foods, including whole grains, fruits and vegetables, high-fiber foods, and high-folate foods.
- Emphasize low glycemic load foods. Check a glycemic load chart to review your current diet and evaluate other, acceptable substitutes with lower glycemic loads.
- Limit your intake of high-fructose corn syrup. Check food labels and do not buy items that contain high-fructose corn syrup.

——— ◆•◆ ———

Chapter 8

Mind–Body Approaches
to a Healthy Heart

The American Institute of Stress estimates that at least 75 percent of visits to primary care physicians are for illnesses caused or worsened by stress. Surprising? Hardly. Most of us are wired: We're on call 24/7, available by telephone, cell phone, and e-mail; we tune in to around-the-clock coverage of around-the-world news. We're slaves to our digital "time-savers," frustrated by rush-hour traffic, and generally in a hurry, overtired, and under *stress*.

When it comes to heart disease, the evidence is clear: Stress plays a major role in triggering heart disease. Many doctors overlook the importance of stress reduction in managing heart disease, but my patients have shown me over the years the damaging effects of excessive stress, as well as the healing influence of mind–body approaches.

The potential of mind–body work for healing heart disease was driven home to me in my work with a fifty-two-year-old urologist who came to see me with high cholesterol and weight management problems. I was able to help him improve his cholesterol somewhat with supplements and low-dose medication, but side effects prevented us from pushing further and he hadn't been able to lose much weight. Frustrated after several months of this plateau, I made my first referral ever to a biofeedback specialist to help him with stress management.

Four months later he came to my office, and I almost didn't recognize him: He had lost twenty-five pounds, his cholesterol had dropped significantly, he had more energy, and he seemed more content with his life overall. I now recommend biofeedback—which includes controlled breathing and progressive muscle relaxation—to many of my patients for help in stress management.

In my practice, most patients are enthusiastic about the idea of mind–body approaches to stress management, although some are skeptical. Some of the more wary patients reconsider when I tell them that I myself do breathing exercises regularly, and I enjoy the rejuvenation I experience after sessions with other mind–body approaches, including healing touch and Reiki. I believe stress reduction is an essential part of good overall health, and what's good for the patient is good for the doctor.

THE LINK BETWEEN STRESS AND CARDIOVASCULAR DISEASE

Since the mid-1970s, a number of studies have emphasized the importance of the mind–body connection, or the link between the brain (thoughts) and the physical response of the nervous system. Scientists now better understand the delicate hormonal and neurological relationships between the mind and the body, particularly in relation to the cardiovascular system.

When faced with stress, the body kicks into the so-called fight-or-flight response, which involves a number of biochemical changes that happen in preparation for dealing with danger. In evolutionary terms, this high-intensity state made sense when quick bursts of energy were required to fight off predators or flee a dangerous situation. Of course, in our daily lives we face fewer actual life-or-death threats, but the modern world remains full of other less intense but more chronic stressors, including financial worries, deadline pressures, and thorny relationships. When confronted with these perceived stressors, our bodies respond in much the same way as our prehistoric ancestors once did.

In the body, all stressors—whether encounters with wild lions or run-ins with wild rush-hour drivers—trigger an alarm in the hypothalamus in the midbrain. The hypothalamus then shifts into overdrive, warning the body that it must prepare for an emergency. As a result, your heart races, breathing hastens, muscles tense, and your metabolism kicks into high gear. You're ready for action. As part of the intricate system of stress response, your body releases adrenaline (which raises blood pressure and heart rate) and other factors that lead to increased inflammation (CRP) and elevated cholesterol. While not harmful in short bursts, this well-orchestrated stress response can cause serious health problems if the stress persists.

In fact, the INTERHEART study concluded that psychosocial stresses—hostility, depression, anxiety, and a sense of hopelessness—account for about 30 percent of the risk of developing a heart attack. Fortunately, the study also concluded that stress can be reversed with social support, regular exercise, stress reduction training, a sense of humor, optimism, charitable work, faith, and pet ownership.

THE LINK BETWEEN STRESS AND ELEVATED CHOLESTEROL

Although the relationship between stress and cholesterol is seldom appreciated, I often observe this connection in my practice. Patients involved in difficult job situations, rocky marriages, or other life crises frequently experience profound jumps in their cholesterol levels, despite no apparent changes in diet or exercise.

Fortunately, the stress response can be quickly reversed. Your body begins to relax as soon as your brain receives the signal that the danger has passed and it's safe to calm down. Within seconds after the brain cancels the emergency signals to the central nervous system, the panic messages cease and relaxation begins. Your heart rate and breathing gradually slow down, and your other systems return to their normal levels.

Now that you understand the influence of stress on your heart health, I encourage you to harness the power of this approach to help you lower your blood pressure and reduce your cholesterol. We will explore the mind–body techniques I have found to be the most useful in my own practice, including biofeedback, energy therapies, massage, and meditation.

BIOFEEDBACK

Biofeedback involves training yourself to use your mind to voluntarily control your body's internal systems. The technique has been successfully used to treat high blood pressure and heart failure and to assist in stroke rehabilitation, among other applications. The beauty of biofeedback is that it allows you to learn about your own body, and how best to tune the relaxation techniques to your particular needs. During biofeedback sessions, various relaxation techniques are practiced while monitoring your body's response—often with visual displays on a computer screen—including heart rate, blood pressure, and muscle tension. Using this information, you can literally watch yourself relax—or become more tense.

As Dr. Andrew Weil points out in his highly recommended audio book *Breathing: The Master Key to Self Healing,* breathing is the only bodily function that can be performed entirely voluntarily (for example, when you intentionally hyperventilate) or entirely involuntarily (as in sleep) using the involuntary or autonomic nervous system. When we practice breathing techniques for relaxation (slow, regular breathing from the abdomen rather than the chest), we are able to gain access to the involuntary nervous system, and influence it to release the stranglehold it often exerts to raise blood pressure, heart rate, and cholesterol. Biofeedback is simply a means for monitoring the impact of breath work and other relaxation techniques.

You can actually learn to control your body's internal processes by carefully studying the measurable changes in your body as you relax and change your breathing, muscle tension, or thought patterns. Once you learn to adjust your physical state to promote relaxation, you can do it without all the equipment.

If you would like to try biofeedback as an addition to your prevention program, I recommend that you locate a professional certified by the Biofeedback Certification Institute of America (www.bcia.org; 10200 West 44th Avenue, Suite 310, Wheat Ridge, CO 80033; 303-420-2902). Ask your physician for a referral. Before making an appointment, also inquire about fees and find out whether the training will be covered by your health insurance plan.

ENERGY THERAPIES (HEALING TOUCH, REIKI)

Only a few years ago, I could never have imagined that I would be recommending energy therapies, including healing touch and Reiki. My initial skepticism is probably understandable, since these treatments were never mentioned in my formal medical training. What's more, the underlying concept is abstract: the idea that every living being emanates an energy field that can be manipulated by a trained practitioner to promote health. But here again, my patients have served as my teachers in showing me how effective energy work can be for stress reduction, pain management, and an overall sense of rejuvenation. I have received several such treatments myself and can attest to the sense of complete refreshment I experienced afterward at the end of a long, busy day.

Healing touch and Reiki are both energy therapies that promote healing and relaxation. Healing touch is intended to support the individual's energy system by activating various energy centers in the body with hand motions intended to smooth any disruptions in an individual's energy field. The technique is practiced by nurses and other health care professionals, as well as laypeople who have been trained in the approach.

Reiki is a Japanese approach to healing that is based on the concept that an unseen life force energy flows through all living things and can be shared. The technique focuses on the whole person—body, mind, spirit, and emotions—creating feelings of relaxation, peace, and well-being. The treatment also involves a commitment to self-improvement. Reiki classes are taught nationwide.

For more information, contact:

- Healing Touch International: www.healingtouchinternational.org; 445 Union Boulevard, Suite 105, Lakewood, CO 80228; 303-989-7982.
- International Association of Reiki Professionals: www.iarp.org; P.O. Box 6182, Nashua, NH 03063; 603-881-8838.

MASSAGE

Massage is much more than a way to ease muscle pain; it is also a powerful mind–body tool for stress management. Massage loosens the autonomic grip on your nervous system to lower your heart rate and decrease blood pressure. Studies have shown that it reduces anxiety and stress-related hormones and, as opposed to medication, heightens your level of alertness instead of making you feel drowsy.

I highly recommend considering massage therapy as a piece of your stress reduction program. Most states require licensing of massage therapists; if your state doesn't, look for a therapist with certification from a professional organization.

For information on state licensing requirements and a list of certified massage therapists in your area, contact:

- National Certification Board for Therapeutic Massage and Bodywork: www.ncbtmb.com; 1901 Meyers Road, Suite 240, Oakbrook Terrace, IL 60181; 630-627-8000.
- American Massage Therapy Association: www.amta-massage.org; 500 Davis Street, Suite 900, Evanston, IL 60201; 708-905-2700; 877-905-2700.

MEDITATION

Though it comes in many different forms or traditions, meditation typically involves focusing your complete attention on one thing at a time. Focus is usually aided by concentrating on a word or belief that has special meaning to you. Because we are most accustomed to our minds being full of thoughts and memories, most people initially find this focused attention to be difficult. It can be a real challenge to maintain concentration when faced with a barrage of distracting thoughts.

I invite you to try it now. Put this book down, sit in a comfortable position with your eyes closed, and try to sweep your mind clear of any image or thought. If a problem comes to your attention, try to banish it so that your mind is completely clear. Initially, it might only be possible to maintain this kind of concentration for a minute or two. Strangely, it takes practice to be able to think about absolutely nothing.

Meditation relieves stress because it is impossible to feel tense or angry when your mind is focused somewhere else. You can't experience negative thoughts—or the physiological responses to those thoughts—if your mind is tuned in to a neutral stimulus.

Studies back up the idea that meditation promotes relaxation. Research dating back to 1968 at Harvard Medical School found that when people practiced Transcendental Meditation (TM, a type of mantra meditation), they showed physiological signs of deep relaxation: They experienced a dramatic reduction in heart rate and blood pressure, as well as a decrease in the amount of oxygen required to maintain normal functioning. Learning to meditate could actually help your body reverse the process of hardening of the arteries, according to a study published in *Stroke,* a journal of the American Heart

Association. Sixty men and women with high blood pressure were assigned to either a Transcendental Meditation program or a control group. The meditation group practiced twenty minutes twice a day. After seven months, those practicing TM showed a surprising reduction in the level of plaque, reducing their overall heart attack risk up to 11 percent and their stroke risk up to 15 percent. The other group had no improvement; in fact, their plaque levels increased.

Another study found that when it comes to reducing atherosclerosis, the overall effectiveness of a program that involved meditation and yoga along with a high-fiber, low-fat diet, aerobic exercise, and antioxidant supplements was even greater than in studies involving cholesterol-lowering drugs.

For more information about meditation, contact:

- Cambridge Insight Meditation Center: www.cimc.info; 331 Broadway, Cambridge, MA 02139; 617-441-9038.
- The Mind/Body Medical Institute: www.mbmi.org; 824 Boylston Street, Chestnut Hill, MA 02467; 617-991-0102.
- The Center for Mindfulness in Medicine, Health Care, and Society (University of Massachusetts Medical Center): www.umassmed.edu/cfm; 55 Lake Avenue North, Worcester, MA 01655; 508-856-2656.

YOGA

Yoga promotes a deep sense of relaxation while at the same time lowering blood pressure and reducing cholesterol. These health benefits make yoga an ideal tool in promoting cardiovascular health.

Yoga combines deep breathing with systematically moving

the body into a series of postures, or positions. Classes for beginners can be very gentle and noncompetitive, making it an ideal exercise for people who have grown out of shape over the years. But some yoga postures require significant endurance, strength, and flexibility. Since it works every muscle group, weaknesses can be identified easily, allowing you to target areas that need special attention. If you have not exercised in a while, be sure to choose a class for first-time students.

Ancient Sanskrit text describe several types of yoga, including bhakti yoga (emphasis on spirituality), jnana yoga (emphasis on wisdom), karma yoga (emphasis on service), raja yoga (emphasis on concentration), dhyana yoga (emphasis on meditation), mantra yoga (emphasis on reciting sacred words), and hatha yoga (emphasis on energies of the body).

Evidence indicates that yoga can help lower cholesterol and control blood sugar levels. A study of ninety-eight people who participated in an eight-day lifestyle modification program based on yoga found that fasting glucose, total cholesterol, LDL cholesterol, and triglyceride levels were significantly lower and HDL cholesterol levels higher on the last day of the course than the first day. The higher the participant's cholesterol or blood sugar level, the more significant the change.

For background on yoga postures and practicing the technique, check out a book or video on yoga from your local library or take a class. For more information, contact:

- Integral Yoga Institute: www.integralyogany.org; 227 West 13th Street, New York, NY 10011; 212-929-0586.
- www.yogafinder.com provides an online guide to yoga classes nationwide.

THE HEALING POWER OF FAITH

Studies of the effect of spiritual and religious beliefs on cardiovascular health have consistently shown that a spiritual belief system helps maintain good health. In one study of adults over age sixty, those who attended religious services were less likely to have been admitted to the hospital within the previous year and, if admitted, spent fewer days in the hospital than those who did not attend services. Another study found that prayer and regular participation in religious services were associated with a significant reduction in blood pressure.

TAKE THIS TO HEART

- The link between stress and cholesterol is vastly underrecognized.
- Stress management and relaxation techniques should be considered an integral piece of a complete heart disease prevention program. I have found particular value in biofeedback, energy therapies (healing touch, Reiki), massage, meditation, yoga, and spiritual practices.

— • ◆ • —

Chapter 9

Exercise

When it comes to your cardiovascular health, you can be a more powerful healer than your doctor. Whenever I prescribe a supplement or medication, I always tell my patients that the pills are only half of what they need; the other half comes from what they can do on their own—exercise and dietary changes. To drive home this message, I often remark to my patients: "Dr. Devries has done his part; now it is up to you to be the doctor and begin the most powerful treatment—exercise."

When it comes to exercise, you can write your own prescription. You need enough regular exercise to protect against cardiovascular disease, but you can choose the type of activity, when to do it, and how long to do it at any one time. Good news (especially if you don't like to exercise): Small amounts of exercise add up to big changes in cardiovascular health.

For me, finding time to exercise is probably the most difficult part of my health care. My routine demands that I wake up at 4:45 AM, and I simply can't get up earlier to make time to exercise. (Sleep is important to health, too.) Instead, I try to work out after dinner with my children; this gives us time together, and creates a routine that benefits our entire family.

In this chapter, you will find some surprising and powerful data about exercise, as well as practical tips to help you launch your own exercise program.

EXERCISE AND CARDIOVASCULAR DISEASE

You undoubtedly know that physical activity is good for your health, but you may not fully appreciate the medicinal power of exercise. A study in the *Journal of the American Medical Association* examined the exercise habits of 44,500 men from 1986 to 1998. The study found that compared with men who did not exercise:

- Men who ran for one hour or more per week had 42 percent fewer heart attacks.
- Those who trained with weights for thirty minutes or more per week had 23 percent fewer heart attacks.
- Those who rowed for one hour or more per week had 18 percent fewer heart attacks.
- Those who walked briskly for half an hour per day had 18 percent fewer heart attacks.

While that study reviewed the effect of exercise on heart attack risk, exercise can do much more:

- Reduce your risk of developing certain cancers.
- Minimize your risk of developing colds and respiratory infections.
- Relieve anxiety, stress, and depression.
- Improve mental alertness, memory, and sexual desire.

- Reduce arthritis pain.
- Improve flexibility.

In fact, if all the benefits of exercise could be extracted into a pill, its value would make it far too expensive for any of us to afford!

You don't have to spend hours in the gym to enjoy the benefits of exercise. Studies have shown that as little as thirty minutes a day of light physical activity will reduce your risk of disease by lowering blood pressure and cholesterol. That's physical activity, not hard-core exercise. This is even easier knowing that you don't have to do your entire exercise routine in a single shot; breaking up your workout into two fifteen-minute sessions—one in the beginning and the other at the end of your day—is a great solution for many people who find it easier to carve out shorter periods of exercise. Divided exercise sessions work particularly well for walkers, who can get up and go without the need for changing clothes or preparation.

Of course, these studies looked at minimum levels of exercise. To maximize your benefit, you'll want to go harder and longer. But the point is that with even a nominal level of exertion, you can enjoy a major turnabout in your overall health.

Similar to treatment with medicine, benefits continue only while you remain active and are quickly lost once you stop taking your exercise medicine. For example, a 2003 study involved people who went through an eight-month training program consisting of two strength training and two aerobic training sessions per week. These subjects experienced many benefits in their cholesterol profile, including a 9 mg/dL reduction in total cholesterol, an 18 mg/dL drop in triglyceride level, and a 5 mg/dL increase in HDL. All of these benefits melted away after exercise was stopped for three months.

One study found that those who had already suffered a heart attack reduced their risk of a second attack by 20 to 25 percent when they started to exercise. These heart-saving benefits show up after as little as six to ten weeks of regular aerobic exercise.

The bottom line: Exercise is great medicine. Write yourself a prescription for regular use with unlimited refills!

A well-rounded exercise program includes three components: aerobic conditioning, strength training, and stretching. While you won't necessarily do all types of exercise during every workout, your weekly routine should include all three.

AEROBIC CONDITIONING

The term *aerobic* means "using oxygen." During aerobic exercise, large muscles in your body are active for an extended period of time, requiring a rush of oxygen and a fast heartbeat. The more of this kind of workout you do, the more efficient your entire body becomes: Your heart, like any muscle, becomes stronger and the muscles in your legs become more efficient at doing work with less oxygen.

Most people think of aerobic exercise as activity that requires gym equipment, such as a treadmill, elliptical machine, ski machine, or rowing simulator. Although these provide a great workout (personally, I prefer the elliptical machine when exercising indoors), a health-club-type workout is certainly not essential. Other highly effective aerobic activities that can be done outside a gym include recreational walking, jogging, bicycling, or swimming.

These activities share the common theme of requiring rhythmic, repeated use of the major muscle groups. When done regularly—three times a week for at least twenty minutes—aerobic activities improve the efficiency of the heart, lungs, and muscles and increase their ability to be more active with less stress to your body.

For maximum benefit, you need to work hard enough—but it is possible to go overboard. Cardiovascular conditioning takes place when your heart beats at 70 to 85 percent of its maximum safe rate. Your maximum heart rate is approximately 220 minus your age. (See the following table.) Check your pulse before starting to exercise, every few minutes during exercise, and immediately after stopping.

Measure your heart rate at the radial artery; you can find it by extending your arm with your palm up and feeling on the thumb side of your wrist. Using a watch, count your pulse for ten seconds, then multiply that number by 6 to get the number of beats per minute. During exercise, a pulse that is under your target range indicates you may need to speed up or work harder, while one that is higher means that you should slow down.

Target Pulse Ranges

Age	Maximum Heart Rate	Target Range
30	190	133–162
35	185	130–157
40	180	126–153
45	175	122–140
50	170	119–145
55	165	115–140
60	160	112–136
65	155	109–132

Target Pulse Ranges (*continued*)

Age	Maximum Heart Rate	Target Range
70	150	105–128
75	145	102–123
80	140	98–119

The target heart rates above are only guidelines. As a general rule, you should be able to comfortably carry on a conversation while you are working out. If you feel as if the exercise you are doing is so easy that you could continue indefinitely without much effort, the intensity is probably too low. On the other hand, if exercise leaves you gasping for breath and you cannot continue for at least twenty minutes, the intensity of your workout needs to be ratcheted down.

If you're new to exercise, start slow. Try ten minutes of light to moderate exercise three times a week and gradually extend your workout time to twenty or thirty minutes, then increase the intensity.

Aim for workouts of moderate intensity—about 70 to 85 percent of your maximum heart rate. If you work at the higher end of the exercise benefit zone, you will experience a faster improvement in your athletic ability, but this extra effort could increase your risk of injury. The death rate from cardiovascular disease is much lower in moderate exercisers than in nonexercisers, but only slightly lower in heavy exercisers. In addition, moderate exercise reduces stress, anxiety, and blood pressure as effectively as strenuous exercise does.

You can monitor the improvement in your physical conditioning by checking your pulse. As your body becomes more efficient, you will notice that your resting heart rate gradually slows. Over time, you will also find that it takes more exercise to increase your pulse to the same level that you used to reach after a short time. The reasons are that exercise strengthens your heart, and that your body requires less oxygen.

Remember to add an "appetizer" before your workout and a "dessert" afterward with a five-minute warm-up and cool-down consisting of very low-intensity exercise. A good idea for a warm-up is to go through the motions of the main workout at a slower pace. For your cool-down, walk slowly for three to five minutes, or until your heart rate returns close to your starting point.

Tips for Varying Aerobic Workouts

- Use the equipment in a different way. If you exercise in an area with more than one kind of machine, switch to a different piece of equipment every five to ten minutes. This change-up will add variety and make your workout more interesting. I usually switch from an elliptical to a rowing machine, then to a treadmill—all in a single thirty-minute session!
- Change the way you use the equipment. For example, I like to reverse the direction of the elliptical platform every few minutes or reverse the direction of pedaling on a stationary bicycle.
- Frequently change the intensity of your workout. Intense bursts requiring high energy strengthen your heart and help build muscle.

STRENGTH TRAINING

Most people barely realize that, over the years, they are slowly losing muscle mass and strength. Fortunately, strength training can completely reverse this process. The typical American loses 10 to 20 percent of muscle strength between the ages of twenty and fifty, and then another 25 to 30 percent between fifty and seventy. In addition, every decade from age forty on, the average person loses six pounds of muscle; this change in body composition from muscle to fat can change the shape of your body even if it doesn't change your weight on the scales, because muscle is denser than fat.

Strength Training Builds Muscle and Melts Fat

In addition to making you stronger, strength training can help you lose weight. Muscle is one of the most metabolically active tissues in your body. The greater your muscle mass, the hotter you run your body's metabolic furnace (or metabolic rate) and the easier it is to slim down. At age twenty, the average woman has 23 percent body fat; the average man, 19 percent. At thirty-five those fat figures have jumped to 30 percent and 25 percent, respectively. And by age sixty, the average woman's body is 44 percent fat, and the average man's, 38 percent. The increase in body fat directly corresponds to a decrease in muscle mass over the years.

To halt this shift from muscle to fat, it is important to put together a balanced exercise program, including both aerobics and strength-building exercises. People who do aerobics but skip the weight training still lose muscle mass and gain fat— about one pound of muscle every two years after age twenty.

In fact, regular strength training can, in some ways, turn

back the aging process when it comes to muscles. For example, one study found that seventy-year-old men who had performed strength training since middle age were just as strong, on average, as twenty-eight-year-old men who didn't strength train!

What an uplifting message: You're never too old to grow stronger. And the more out of shape you are, the greater your opportunity. Frail octogenarians can easily double or triple their strength in just a couple of months. One study found that ninety-year-old nursing home residents increased their muscle strength by up to 180 percent in an eight-week exercise program. Imagine what a difference this added strength could make in maintaining independence in the elderly.

The specific exercises that would be included in a strength training program go beyond the material that we can cover in this book. I recommend that you take a class at a local health club or community center or pick up an exercise book or video from the library or bookstore. A wide range of simple, inexpensive programs are available whether you choose to work out at home or at a gym.

STRETCHING

Remember back to the days you could easily touch your toes or maybe even do the splits? Most of us tighten up over time, leading to poor posture, back problems, and a limited range of motion in our arms and legs. Flexibility is a critical component of fitness, but one that is often overlooked. Without regular stretching, the average adult's flexibility declines by 5 percent per decade. The only way to preserve your flexibility is to add stretching exercises to your exercise program.

As little as ten minutes of stretching every other day can help to prevent stiffness and loss of flexibility. Your stretch will be more effective and you will feel better if your muscles are warmed up when you start. To build flexibility, bend or flex until you feel tension or slight discomfort—but not pain—and hold each stretch for about thirty seconds. Try not to hold your breath or bounce while stretching in order to avoid tearing the connective tissue in your joints.

Building strength and increasing flexibility are not mutually exclusive—in fact, they are both critical to maintaining optimal conditioning. I recommend that you pick up a book (an excellent resource with easy-to-follow diagrams is Paul Chek's *How to Eat, Move and Be Healthy!*) or try a class at a local gym or recreation facility. Once you learn the components of a good, basic stretching routine, you can follow them wherever you work out.

HOME VERSUS AWAY: PLANNING YOUR EXERCISE PROGRAM

Whether you exercise at a top-of-the-line health club or a corner of your unfinished basement, a good exercise program includes the same basic ingredients:

Monday (Aerobic Workout)

5 minutes: Stretching/warm-up
30 minutes: Aerobics

Health Club Options	At-Home Options
Treadmill	Fast walking
Exercise bike	Jogging
Elliptical machine	Bicycling
Swimming	Home equipment
Aerobics class	Exercise video

5 minutes: Stretching/cool-down

> ### Tuesday (Strength Training)
>
> 5 minutes: Stretching/warm-up
> 30 minutes: Strength training
>
> | ***Health Club Options*** | ***At-Home Options*** |
> |---|---|
> | **Free weights** | **Free weights** |
> | **Weight machines** | **Pilates video** |
> | **Pilates** | |
>
> 5 minutes: Stretching/cool-down
>
> ### Wednesday (Aerobic Workout) Repeat
> ### Thursday (Strength Training) Repeat
> ### Friday (Aerobic Training) Repeat
> ### Saturday (Strength Training) Repeat
> ### Sunday—Rest

GETTING STARTED

I know how hard it is to exercise regularly; maintaining a consistent exercise program remains a personal challenge for me. For most people, exercise is something that is not considered a priority, but will get done "if time allows." This approach is almost certainly doomed to failure, as no one has enough time in their day. I always invite patients to think of their lack of exercise as the result of making exercise a low priority. I remind them (and myself) that if they were paid five hundred dollars for each exercise session, most people would exercise every day without fail. The bottom line is: If you believe that exercise is important enough, you will make the time.

Mental Exercises to Get You on the Exercise Track

- Think back to a time in the past when you exercised regularly. What was different then that allowed you to exercise compared with now? Is it possible to re-create some of the circumstances that allowed you to exercise more consistently in the past?
- Schedule exercise into your week. Plan ahead and make exercise an appointment on your daily calendar.
- Try to exercise with someone to help keep both of you motivated. If this is not practical, set up a friendly competition with someone else and compare the frequency of your workouts.
- Savor the energized feeling you experience immediately after exercise and concentrate on how wonderful it would be to feel that way more often.

One year of regular exercise can return your body to a level of fitness it enjoyed ten years ago. Try finding a pill to pull off that kind of miracle!

TAKE THIS TO HEART

- Remember that you have the potential to be a powerful healer. Only you can implement an exercise program—a therapy more potent than pills.
- If you really believe in your heart that exercise is a high priority, you will make the time to do it regularly.
- Design your exercise program to include at least twenty minutes of aerobic exercise every other

day; strength training on alternate days; and stretching before and after your aerobic workouts.

- Consult your doctor before starting an exercise program; a stress test might be needed before you can safely begin, especially if you have risk factors for heart disease.

Chapter 10

Quitting Smoking

My patients are my greatest teachers, and one patient who taught me a great deal was a vibrant, well-read woman in her fifties who came to see me for help in developing a heart disease prevention program. She proudly announced that she had recently quit smoking after more than two decades of futile attempts. Ultimately, she found success with biofeedback and medical hypnosis. Her victory, against all odds, motivated me to explore the role of mind–body approaches to smoking cessation.

About 70 percent of the forty-eight million American smokers say they want to quit. When they ask for help from their doctors, most physicians recommend nicotine gum and patches or write out a prescription for a smoking cessation drug. In my opinion, too few doctors suggest that their patients try medical hypnosis, biofeedback, and other mind–body techniques.

I find mind–body approaches to be, by far, the most effective tool available for smoking cessation, largely because they address both the physical and psychological obstacles to quitting.

In my practice, I refer patients who wish to stop smoking to experts in biofeedback and medical hypnosis first, turning to medication if a patient needs additional support.

SMOKING AND CARDIOVASCULAR DISEASE

Smoking is the greatest preventable risk to your health. In addition to causing emphysema and lung cancer, it may surprise you to learn that smoking is presumed responsible for about one of every three deaths from heart disease. These are a few of the ways smoking ravages the heart and circulatory system:

- Smoking lowers levels of the protective HDL cholesterol by up to 4 mg/dL in men and 6 mg/dL in women. This translates into an 8 percent increase in cardiac risk for men and a whopping 18 percent greater risk for women.
- Smoking damages the blood vessels, making them less elastic, leading to high blood pressure.
- Smoking stimulates the development of blood clots.
- Smoking starves the body of oxygen by forcing carbon monoxide to fill places in the blood usually reserved for oxygen.
- Smoking damages the lining of the arteries, causing inflammation and high levels of C-reactive protein.

While nicotine stands out as the best-known toxin in cigarettes, smoke also contains carbon monoxide, hydrogen cyanide, arsenic, lead, cadmium, dioxin, and at least four thousand other toxic chemicals. In addition, cigarette smoke includes a significant amount of radioactive materials. It has been estimated that someone who smokes a pack and a half of cigarettes a day is exposed to a dose of radiation equal to about three hundred chest X-rays per year!

Your risk might be increased by the company you keep: Secondhand smoke is a potent toxin to your heart. According to the American Heart Association, approximately thirty-seven to forty thousand nonsmokers die each year from cardiovascular disease resulting from passive exposure to tobacco smoke. The potent effects of secondhand smoke were highlighted in a study in Helena, Montana, where the risk of heart disease dropped precipitously once public smoking was banned.

Don't assume that cigars are safer than cigarettes even though cigar smokers don't inhale. A study of 17,774 men found that cigar smokers were more likely to develop cardiovascular disease than nonsmokers, and twice as likely as nonsmokers to suffer from cancer of the mouth, throat, and lungs.

Cigar smoking causes almost twice as many heart attacks and strokes as it does lung cancer. Why? Because cigars can have more than twenty times as much nicotine as the average cigarette.

A BREATH OF GOOD NEWS

Fortunately, the body works tirelessly to heal itself as soon as you quit smoking. According to a 1990 Surgeon General's Report, *The Health Benefits of Smoking Cessation,* quitting smoking reduces the risk of death from heart disease by 50 percent or more. Within twenty minutes of your last cigarette, the nicotine in your bloodstream begins to wane and your blood vessels begin to relax. In response, your blood pressure drops, your heart rate slows, and your overall circulation improves. Within eight hours of your last cigarette, carbon monoxide levels drop in the bloodstream and oxygen levels increase.

Within two weeks of quitting smoking, you can expect a significant boost in the level of your good HDL cholesterol. When you've been smoke-free for six months, your HDL cholesterol increases to your pre-smoking level. By the time you reach your one-year anniversary as a nonsmoker, your risk of heart attack is reduced by 50 percent.

Quitting adds years to your life. Men who quit between the ages of thirty-five and thirty-nine add an average of five years to their lives, while women in the same age group add three years. Some people are not motivated by the prospect of increased longevity promised by smoking cessation; "I would rather smoke and be happy than live a few extra months," they say. My point is that the ravages of smoking, including stroke, heart failure, and cancer, often leave afflicted patients wishing for a shorter life.

Fortunately, in my practice, I see long-term smokers quit on a regular basis. The key question to ask is: Are you convinced that you want to stop smoking? If you are not absolutely certain that you are ready to quit, there is no sense in pursuing methods to help you, as they will certainly not work. If, on the other hand, the answer is unequivocally yes, review the information below and check out the Internet references provided. Discuss the information with your doctor to devise a strategy best suited for your specific needs.

MIND–BODY APPROACHES TO SMOKING CESSATION

Mind–body approaches are so successful because they address both the physical and psychological aspects of addiction. Mind–body approaches focus on the vast power of your mind to quash the body's physical responses to nicotine withdrawal.

I have found these techniques to be of great value and, best of all, without side effects of any kind.

Medical hypnosis is a mind–body technique in which thoughts of the damage smoking inflicts and the sense of well-being expected after quitting are communicated while the individual is in a particularly receptive state. These suggestions are often paired with biofeedback techniques to control the physical aspects of addiction. Those who use medical hypnosis are three times as likely to quit smoking as those relying on willpower alone. A review of fifty-nine studies on smoking cessation and hypnosis found that many reported a success rate of 50 percent or higher, and those who quit experience a remarkable one-year smoke-free rate of 63 to 88 percent.

MEDICAL AIDS TO STOP SMOKING

Some people benefit from various smoking cessation aids.

Nicotine Patch

Over-the-counter nicotine patches attach to the skin and release a dose of nicotine into the bloodstream over time. Products come in two- or three-step programs, so that smokers can gradually reduce their nicotine exposure over a period of eight to sixteen weeks. Instructions on exactly how to use the patch are provided with each package. Studies have shown that the successful quit rate is higher with the patch than quitting cold turkey. In addition, it appears that people who use the patch gain less weight as they quit.

Nicotine Gum

Over-the-counter nicotine gum is available in 2- and 4-milligram doses. The gum comes with instructions, but many people use it improperly. It works by allowing you to absorb nicotine through your gums, so it needs to be in contact with them. After chewing for about twenty seconds or so, slip the gum between your cheek and gums, where the nicotine will be easily absorbed.

Medication

Many smokers find success in quitting with the support of the short-term use of Zyban (bupropion). It can be used alone or in combination with nicotine replacement. Zyban is a two-month prescription; for the first week, the patient takes the drug while continuing to smoke. After a week, the medication has reached an effective level in the body, blunting the physical symptoms of addiction. At that point, the patient can quit cold turkey without suffering the physical symptoms of nicotine withdrawal. While the drug has been very successful, it should not be used by people with seizure disorders, and interactions with other medications can limit its use.

Studies have shown that medication can be very effective. A study published in the *New England Journal of Medicine* examined the effectiveness of Zyban alone, the nicotine patch alone, or the two in combination, as compared with a placebo (sugar pills plus an inactive patch) in 893 smokers. All participants received counseling and supportive phone calls throughout the twelve-month study. At the end of the study, the quit rate was 5.6 percent in the placebo group, 9.8 percent in the patch group, 18.4 percent in the Zyban alone group, and 22.5 in the combined medication/patch group. People treated with any form of nicotine replacement experienced less weight gain and fewer withdrawal symptoms.

No matter how you do it, quitting smoking is difficult, but it remains one of the most important steps you can take to improve your cardiovascular health.

BEWARE OF OVERDOSE

Do not smoke cigarettes when you are using nicotine replacement products to avoid overdose. The signs of nicotine poisoning include severe headaches, weakness, dizziness, nausea, vomiting, diarrhea, cold sweats, blurred vision, hearing difficulties, and mental confusion. If you develop any of these symptoms, contact your physician immediately.

WHERE TO GET HELP

- www.smokefree.gov: In addition to online information, this government-sponsored site offers online and telephone support.
- www.americanheart.org: This American Heart Association Web site provides information on quitting; search under "smoking cessation."
- www.lungusa.org: This American Lung Association Web site includes a section titled "Freedom from Smoking."
- www.cancer.org: The American Cancer Society site

provides information on quitting; search under "quitting smoking."

TAKE THIS TO HEART

- If you smoke, quitting is the most important single step you can take to reduce your risk of a heart attack.
- First consider mind–body approaches to smoking cessation, including medical hypnosis and biofeedback.
- Other useful tools to help you quit smoking include short-term use of the prescription medication Zyban or nicotine replacement products.

Chapter 11

When to Consider Medication for Cholesterol Treatment

Note: This section is provided for background information only; it is not intended to be used as medical advice. Do not make any changes in your use of supplements or prescription medications without the approval of your physician. Some of the use of medication described in this chapter is based on my own clinical experience, but it is not contained in the manufacturer's prescribing information.

My patients tend to be health-conscious, goal-oriented people who want to optimize their cholesterol and reduce their cardiac risks in the safest way possible. For many, that means avoiding prescription medications, especially statins. One patient pleaded with me: "Doc, whatever you do, don't put me on those 'Satan' medicines."

While I applaud my patients' efforts to seek safe and natural treatments for their cardiovascular challenges, there are times when prescription medications are necessary. In my opinion, statins and other cardiac medications are safe and beneficial for the vast majority of cardiac patients who take them. For those patients who do not respond adequately to lifestyle changes and supplements, prescription medications can be lifesavers.

That said, I do think that many doctors put too much emphasis on medication, paying little attention to the underlying health issues of diet, exercise, and lifestyle. In my opinion, *everyone* needs to take an honest inventory of their lifestyle choices, making adjustments as necessary. Most of us don't always eat well, exercise often, or rest as much as we should, and generally fail to take care of ourselves as well as we deserve.

Lifestyle changes cannot lower cholesterol levels adequately for everyone. About 20 to 25 percent of the population, by virtue of having been born with the wrong genes, has the biological deck stacked against them. These people may do everything right—maintain a healthy weight, exercise regularly, eat healthy foods—and still have unhealthy cholesterol levels or other metabolic risk factors. They may need prescription medication in order to lower their cholesterol to the desirable range. In addition, people facing additional health risks, including diabetes or vascular disease, are good candidates for medication to lower their cholesterol.

Medication and lifestyle changes are in no way mutually exclusive. When I prescribe medication, I always tell my patients that I am giving them only 50 percent of what they need; the other half comes from their diet and exercise plans. The most disturbing message I sometimes hear from patients is that they have been told that if they go on cholesterol-lowering medication, they don't need to be careful about what they eat. Nothing could be further from the truth. In fact, one study published in the *Journal of the American Medical Association* found that only half of the people relying on cholesterol-lowering medications alone lowered their cholesterol to the target range, while 80 percent of those who used medication *and* dietary changes achieved their cholesterol goals. Maintaining a healthy lifestyle while on cholesterol medication has another bonus: The dose required for excellent results will be much lower than if you rely on the pills alone.

AN OVERVIEW OF COMMON CHOLESTEROL DRUGS

Cholesterol-lowering medications can be an essential part of treatment, especially for high-risk patients or those for whom natural options have not yielded the desired results. This chapter provides a brief overview of common cholesterol-lowering medications; it is not intended to be a comprehensive guide. *Only your doctor can determine which medication is right for you based on your individual medical needs.*

While doctors can choose from among dozens of medications to lower cholesterol and improve lipid profiles, the following is a brief summary of common cholesterol drugs and their uses. These medications have three uses: to lower LDL cholesterol, to raise HDL cholesterol, and to lower triglyceride levels.

STATINS TO LOWER LDL CHOLESTEROL

This class includes Advicor (a combination of lovastatin and niacin), Crestor (rosuvastatin), Lescol (fluvastatin), Lipitor (atorvastatin), Mevacor (lovastatin), Pravachol (pravastatin), Zocor (simvastatin), and Vytorin (a combination of Zetia and Zocor).

- Statins lower LDL cholesterol by as much as 60 percent at high doses.
- Statins reduce inflammation and lower C-reactive protein levels by as much as 40 percent.

How They Work

Statins reduce cholesterol levels by blocking HMG-CoA reductase, a key protein needed by the liver to make cholesterol. Since about 70 percent of cholesterol is manufactured in the liver, the body tries to make up for the production drop by capturing LDL cholesterol from the bloodstream, causing the LDL level in the blood to drop.

All statins work similarly, but they differ slightly in chemical structure, leading to differences in potency and in the way they are cleared from the body. These differences account for variations in side effects from one drug to another; you might experience negative side effects with one statin but not another. In addition, as the chart on page 158 shows, various brands of statins can differ significantly in how effective they are at lowering LDL cholesterol.

Side Effects

While statins are generally very safe, they do have the potential to cause significant unwanted side effects:

• **Liver problems.** The most common concern of patients I see is fear of liver damage from statins. The chance of irritating the liver (very rarely leading to permanent problems) while taking the lowest doses of statins is less than one out of two hundred; at the highest doses, the chance jumps to one out of fifty.

Irritation of the liver does not cause any symptoms; abnormal blood tests of liver function are required to identify the problem. For this reason, it is very important to have blood tests to monitor the liver function before starting statins, several weeks after starting statins, and periodically thereafter. The good news is that when irritation does develop from statins, it resolves in nearly every case once the medicine is stopped. In my practice, I am not aware of a single situation in which a patient became ill from a statin-related liver problem or developed permanent liver disease from the use of statins.

• **Muscle problems.** The issue with statins that I believe is more significant than liver toxicity, although it is not discussed as often, is the effect of the drug on muscles. Fortunately, the most severe side effect—actual muscle breakdown—is rare: about one out of five thousand for those taking the lowest doses and one out of two hundred for those taking the highest doses of statins. Very few people take the highest dose, estimated at less than 1 percent of those on statins. These patients tend to have extremely high cholesterol, so that the benefit of the medicine outweighs the side effects. In my nearly twenty years of experience with patients, I have never seen a single case of actual muscle breakdown.

Less dramatic but nevertheless troublesome side effects on the muscles, including cramping and pain, are much more common. This type of muscle soreness feels different from the everyday aches and pains we all experience from time to time.

Other patients have reported unusual numbness or tingling in the hands and fingers. I have one patient, a bighearted philanthropist in his sixties, who, after having started on a statin, described a new tingling in his hands while riding his motorcycle cross-country. (We discussed the non-statin-related danger of this activity as well!) He switched to another statin, and the problem completely resolved.

Occasionally, the muscle soreness from statins develops slowly and is not immediately obvious as a side effect from the medication. Muscle soreness is often attributed to simply getting old and not recognized as related to the statin. For this reason, it is very important that you take a mental inventory of your body before and during treatment with statins (or any medication) so that you know what sensations are normal for you. Most people experience various muscle aches and pains that come and go; try to take mental stock of these sensations before you start a medication so that you notice any changes. By doing so, you will be better able to identify possible medication-related side effects. Any changes, including those that develop over time, should be considered a potential adverse reaction to medication and discussed with your doctor.

When statins do cause muscle aches or soreness, symptoms generally resolve quickly once the medicine is stopped, usually within a few days.

• **Memory problems.** Other potential side effects of statins include clouded thinking and memory problems. Again, if you notice a change in your memory or clarity of thinking while taking statins, talk to your doctor about taking a trial period off the medication. Ironically, other studies have suggested that the use of statins might help reduce the risk of developing Alzheimer's disease.

Minimizing Side Effects

• **Keep the dose low.** The best way to reduce the risk of side effects from statins is to use the lowest dose possible to get the job done. When lifestyle measures have been exhausted and low doses of statins are inadequate, the usual option is to double the dose. The problem is that the biggest bang from the statin comes from the lowest dose; returns diminish as the dose increases.

Surprisingly, as the dose of any statin is doubled—for example, from 20 to 40 milligrams—the impact is only an additional 7 percent LDL reduction. Unfortunately, the risk of side effects can be much higher when the dosage is increased.

- **Switch brands.** If a patient experiences mild side effects and needs a substantial reduction in cholesterol levels, I often replace one statin with another to see if the second brand causes fewer discomforts. Not all statins are created equal; some people respond much better to one brand than another.

- **Add coenzyme Q10.** Another strategy to help prevent statin-related side effects is adding the supplement coenzyme Q10. There are some data, inconclusive at present, to suggest that this supplement can reduce the chance of statin-related side effects. As discussed in chapter 6, CoQ10 is a chemical needed by the body to produce energy. Statins have been shown to reduce the level of this important compound, possibly leading to statin-related muscle pain. The dose of coenzyme Q10 suggested to replenish levels in those taking statins is 100 to 200 milligrams daily.

Who Should Consider Using Statins

- When LDL reduction of more than 25 percent is required to achieve patients' LDL goal, statins may be needed.
- Diabetics and those with vascular disease (diseased arteries in the heart, neck, or legs) are likely candidates for statins.
- Statins should not be used by those with significant liver disease or by women who are pregnant or could become

pregnant. They have been shown to cause harm to developing fetuses in animal studies.

Drug Interactions

When taken with statins, certain medications can increase the risk of complications. These medications include some other classes of cholesterol medicine, some antibiotics and antifungal medicines, and certain blood-pressure- and heart-rhythm-controlling medicines. For this reason, make sure that all your health care providers know about every medicine and supplement you take to avoid prescribing drugs that are likely to clash with one another.

An interesting interaction relates to statins and grapefruit or grapefruit juice. Grapefruit contains a natural blocking substance that makes it difficult for your body to process certain statins, especially Lipitor and Zocor. A grapefruit a day or glass of grapefruit juice should not cause a significant interaction for most people, but avoid drinking more than a quart of grapefruit juice per day while taking a statin medication.

STATINS: CONSIDER THE EVIDENCE

Statins are the most commonly prescribed class of drugs to lower cholesterol. Since they were introduced in 1987, a number of well-designed long-term, randomized clinical trials have consistently shown a reduction in death from cardiovascular disease of about one-third.

- Statins help people with high cholesterol and heart disease. The landmark study highlighting the benefits of statins was the Scandinavian Simvastatin Survival Study—or 4S—trial. Researchers studied 4,444 men and women with heart disease and high total cholesterol; half of the participants took simvastatin for five years, and half took a placebo. At the end of the study, participants taking the statin experienced a 35 percent drop in LDL levels; those in the placebo group had no change in their cholesterol levels. More importantly, those taking the statin had a 30 percent reduction in deaths and a 34 percent lower chance of having a major coronary event during the study compared with those taking a placebo.

- Statins help people with high cholesterol and no history of heart disease. The West of Scotland Coronary Prevention Study examined 6,595 men with elevated cholesterol, but no other signs of heart disease. Half took pravastatin; half were given a placebo. At the end of the study, those taking the statin lowered their LDL cholesterol by 26 percent and reduced their risk of a major coronary event by 31 percent compared with those taking a placebo.

- Statins help people with normal cholesterol and history of diabetes and heart or vascular disease. The Heart Protection Study, published in the journal *Lancet* in 2002, examined the impact of simvastatin on more than twenty thousand people with diabetes or vascular disease. Regardless of their cholesterol level, half received the statin simvastatin; the rest, a placebo. During the five years of the study, those on the statin had 18 percent fewer cardiac deaths and

24 percent fewer first heart attacks and strokes. Surprisingly, even those who started with a low level of LDL (less than 100) experienced significant benefit from taking a statin.

Comparing the Statins

Many people are aware of different brands of statins from advertisements on television and magazines. While only your doctor can determine which medication may be right for you, the following chart summarizes the cholesterol-lowering power of different medications at high and low doses.

Brand Name	Common Low Dose/ LDL Lowering	Maximum Dose/ LDL Lowering
Statins		
Advicor	20 mg/30%	40 mg/42%
Crestor	10 mg/52%	40 mg/63%
Lescol	20 mg/22%	80 mg/35%
Lipitor	10 mg/39%	80 mg/60%
Mevacor	20 mg/27%	80 mg/42%
Pravachol	20 mg/32%	80 mg/37%
Vytorin (combination)	10 mg Zetia + 20 mg Zocor/52%	10 mg Zetia + 80 mg Zocor/60%
Zocor	20 mg/38%	80 mg/47%
Nonstatins		
WelChol	3.6 g/15%	same
Zetia	10 mg/18%	same

ZETIA (EZETIMIBE) TO LOWER LDL CHOLESTEROL

Zetia works in the digestive tract rather than the liver.

- When taken alone, Zetia lowers LDL cholesterol by about 18 percent.
- When used with a statin, Zetia turbocharges the statin to achieve an additional 25 percent LDL lowering beyond that achieved by the statin alone (similar to the effect that would be achieved by increasing the dose of the statin eightfold).
- Zetia is less likely to irritate the liver than statins, making it a better choice for people with mild liver problems.

How It Works

Zetia is a new class of cholesterol medicine that works in a novel way: Rather than cutting cholesterol production by the liver the way statins do, Zetia reduces the amount of cholesterol absorbed by the digestive tract. Zetia can be used by itself or, more commonly, given together with a statin for added benefit. Because higher doses of statins cause higher risks of side effects, rather than prescribe a higher dose of statins, I often combine a low dose of a statin with the helper medicine Zetia. The combination of a statin with Zetia is particularly effective because it provides a one–two punch by blocking production *and* interfering with absorption of cholesterol.

The drug Vytorin is a combination of Zetia and the statin Zocor in a single pill. I have found Vytorin to be particularly useful for patients referred to me who have not tolerated—or those who would like to avoid—higher doses of statins. The lowest dose of Vytorin—10/10 or 10 milligrams of Zetia and 10 milligrams of Zocor—typically achieves close to a 50 percent reduction in LDL, similar to that traditionally requiring 40 to 80 milligrams of statins when used alone.

Side Effects

Zetia rarely causes side effects, but fatigue, stomach pain, and diarrhea have been reported. It can increase the risk of liver problems when taken with a statin, although still less than that expected with the alternative treatment of higher doses of statins alone.

Who Should Consider Using Zetia

- Zetia may be used along with a statin to achieve further LDL reduction without using higher doses of the statin.
- Zetia may be used without additional medication in people who cannot tolerate statins or those with mild liver problems.

A POWERFUL PAIR:
ZETIA ADDED TO RED YEAST RICE

I often see patients in need of substantial LDL lowering who have not been able to tolerate several prescription statins, usually because of muscle aches. Fortunately, I have found a very useful alternative that, in my experience, does the job when all other approaches have failed: the natural statin red yeast rice in combination with the prescription Zetia.

Red yeast rice is effective by itself in lowering LDL, but its potency is substantially boosted with the helper medicine Zetia. Using this combination, I have often been able to lower LDL by 30 to 55 percent—levels previously requiring potent prescription statins. Best of all, I have found this combination to be very well tolerated in those individuals who could not take any prescription statins.

Another combination for those with previous problems with prescription statins is red yeast rice combined with plant sterols. This is somewhat less potent than the combination with Zetia but does not require a prescription. (For more information on red yeast rice, see chapter 6.) Although red yeast rice is obtained over the counter, it is a form of a statin and, therefore, has the potential to cause the same side effects as prescription statins, although in my experience side effects are less common. I advise anyone taking red yeast rice—whether alone or together with another supplement or prescription—to do so only under a physician's supervision.

WELCHOL (COLESEVELAM) TO LOWER LDL CHOLESTEROL

How It Works

Like Zetia, WelChol works in the digestive tract, but by a different mechanism. WelChol binds the cholesterol-rich bile in the intestine. The cholesterol in this mixture cannot be absorbed back into the bloodstream, and the cholesterol level drops. WelChol is not absorbed into circulation, so it does not cause liver toxicity.

On the downside, WelChol is less potent than other options; it reduces LDL by only about 15 percent. It is also more difficult to take. The usual dose is six large pills a day.

Side Effects

WelChol has several possible unwanted side effects, including heartburn, bloating, diarrhea, and constipation.

Who Should Consider Using WelChol

WelChol may be used when LDL reduction is needed in those who have had adverse reactions to other cholesterol medications and in those with mild liver problems.

PRESCRIPTION NIACIN TO RAISE HDL CHOLESTEROL

This class includes Niaspan (nicotinic acid) and Advicor (a combination of lovastatin and Niaspan).

- It raises HDL by up to 26 percent.
- It lowers triglycerides by up to 35 percent.
- It lowers LDL by up to 17 percent.
- It reduces Lp(a) by up to 27 percent.
- It converts small LDL into the more favorable large, fluffy form.

How It Works

Niacin, available in both over-the-counter and prescription forms, is a cholesterol all-star. It improves almost every dimension of a cholesterol profile. (For information on how it works, see the discussion of over-the-counter niacin in chapter 6.)

Side Effects

• **Flushing.** The major problem with niacin is the annoying—but harmless—side effect of flushing and itching (described in detail in chapter 6). This response can last from several minutes to several hours after taking niacin.

Prescription niacin, Niaspan, is prepared in a novel way that slows its entry into the bloodstream, reducing the risk of flushing. Nevertheless, individual responses vary. For some, flushing is less problematic with over-the-counter niacin than with the prescription form.

• **Blood sugar elevation.** Niacin can cause a small increase in blood sugar levels. (Niacin can be used by diabetics with good sugar control but should be avoided by those whose blood sugar levels are not well regulated.)

• **Others.** Niacin can cause a flaring of gout, and worsening of acid indigestion.

Combination Drug

Advicor is a combination of the statin lovastatin and the prescription form of niacin, Niaspan. Advicor can be an excellent choice for people with more than one cholesterol problem, the most common being high LDL and low HDL. If lifestyle changes and supplements are not enough to correct the issues, statins are often used to treat the high LDL. Unfortunately, statins have only a modest effect on raising HDL. For this reason, the combination of statin with niacin, the most potent HDL-raising agent available, is an ideal way to correct both unhealthy LDL and HDL levels.

Advicor lowers LDL by up to 42 percent, while raising HDL by up to 30 percent and reducing triglycerides by up to 44 percent. In my practice, I also use Advicor to help convert LDL to its larger, less risky form, and to reduce high levels of sticky Lp(a). Side effects of Advicor include those mentioned for statins, as well as those of Niaspan.

Who Should Consider Using Niacin

- Niacin is the best agent available for those who need to raise their HDL and lower their Lp(a). In addition, niacin lowers triglycerides moderately, and has a mild LDL-lowering effect.
- Advicor (combination of lovastatin and Niaspan) is ideal for all the reasons listed above for niacin, with the advantage of much greater LDL reduction.

LOVE YOUR LIVER

All cholesterol-lowering drugs can irritate your liver. Generally, lower doses are less likely to cause problems than higher amounts. This kind of liver irritation rarely causes symptoms, so blood tests are needed to identify liver problems. Ideally, your doctor should perform a blood test of liver function before you start a drug (to establish a baseline level), and then retest six to twelve weeks after starting the medication or increasing the dose. If the blood tests show signs of liver irritation, reducing the dose or stopping the medication is nearly always effective in reversing the problem. Once you are on a stable dose of cholesterol medication, your liver tests should be checked periodically (depending on the dose and other medical conditions), even if you do not show signs of problems.

FIBRATES TO LOWER TRIGLYCERIDES

This class includes fenofibrate (Antara, Lofibra, TriCor, and Triglide) and gemfibrozil (Lopid).

- Fibrates lower triglycerides by up to 55 percent.
- Fibrates raise HDL by 7 to 20 percent.
- They also increase LDL particle size.

How They Work

Fibrates are the most effective agents available to reduce triglycerides. They work by cutting the production and stimulating the breakdown of triglycerides in the liver. An optimal triglyceride level is under 100 mg/dL. I usually consider prescribing fibrates when a patient's triglyceride level exceeds 300 mg/dL after lifestyle changes have been exhausted. Lifestyle changes that drop triglycerides include reducing simple carbohydrates in the diet and adding more aerobic exercise. Diabetics (and pre-diabetics) tend to have high triglycerides that improve when the sugar level is brought under control.

In addition to lowering triglycerides, fibrates convert the

harmful small, dense LDL—which is present in about half of the men and one-third of the women with heart disease—into the less risky fluffy type. Fibrates also raise HDL, but not as effectively as niacin.

Side Effects

- The potential side effects of fibrates include liver and muscle irritation.
- Fibrates can interfere with the blood-thinning medicine Coumadin; you need to have your blood thinning monitored closely if you use these two medications together.

Minimizing Side Effects

When fibrates are taken in combination with statins, the risk of side effects—especially liver and muscle irritation—increases significantly. These are some strategies to improve the safety of combination therapy:

- Some fibrates are safer than others for combination therapy. Fenofibrates (Antara, Lofibra, TriCor, and Triglide) tend to be safer with statins than gemfibrozil (Lopid).

    Always use the lowest dose of fibrate possible. The dose of TriCor usually prescribed is 145 milligrams. When I use TriCor together with a statin, I prefer to use the lowest dose, 48 milligrams. This low dose is consistent with my policy of using the smallest possible dose to get the job done; it also minimizes the risk of side effects.

Who Should Consider Using Fibrates

- Fibrates are a good solution to treat very high triglycerides that do not respond to lifestyle changes or treatment of diabetes.
- Fibrates can be useful in raising HDL in people following a healthy lifestyle who cannot tolerate niacin.

PRESCRIPTION FISH OIL TO LOWER TRIGLYCERIDES

Prescription fish oil is similar to over-the-counter fish oil, although it is typically more concentrated.

How It Works

Fish oil is now available by prescription in the product Omacor. I believe this is an interesting acknowledgment by the pharmaceutical industry of the benefit of omega-3s and may lead to more widespread use of these powerful compounds. (For more information on omega-3 fatty acids, see chapter 6.)

Over-the-counter fish oil works perfectly well and contains the same active ingredients as prescription Omacor. The prescription form, however, is a more concentrated version, and, unlike over-the-counter supplements, its composition is regulated—as with all medications approved by the Food and Drug Administration.

Omacor has been studied in patients with very high triglycerides (500 mg/dL or higher). In these patients, high doses of fish oil—4 grams per day—lowered triglycerides by 45 percent and increased HDL by 9 percent. In these same patients, however, LDL increased by 45 percent.

Side Effects

- The side effects of fish oil, whether taken over the counter or by prescription, include stomach upset and gas.
- Fish oil is a mild blood thinner; it should be discontinued two weeks before surgery and should not be taken in high doses with the blood thinner Coumadin.

Who Should Consider Taking Prescription Fish Oil

Most of my patients take over-the-counter fish oil, but I believe the prescription version is a reasonable alternative for those who feel more comfortable with a prescription product or for those whose health insurance makes this option more economical.

TAKE THIS TO HEART

- Although I prefer to avoid prescription medication whenever possible, I believe in a goal-oriented approach. If lifestyle measures and supplements are not enough to reach cholesterol goals—or when the risk of heart disease is high—prescription medication definitely has a role.
- Different kinds of cholesterol problems require different treatments. There is no single "best" cholesterol medicine; each person's individual situation requires a unique approach. In general, however, the following guidelines can be used when considering medication.

- If your cholesterol problem is limited to high LDL, statins are preferred. Zetia and WelChol are less potent than statins but can be effective in people with liver problems or those who have trouble taking statins. A combination of a statin with Zetia allows maximal LDL lowering at low doses of statin.
- If your cholesterol problem is limited to low HDL, niacin (or Niaspan) is preferred. Fibrates are second best for raising HDL and can be used by people who cannot tolerate niacin, or by diabetics whose sugar levels are not under control (since niacin can raise blood sugar levels further).
- If your cholesterol problem is limited to high triglycerides, fish oil is a great natural option, either over the counter or by prescription (Omacor). Fish oil is less potent than niacin or fibrates, but it is useful as sole treatment for triglycerides under 300 mg/dL or as an addition to fibrates or niacin. Fibrates, especially fenofibrates, are the most potent agents for lowering triglycerides. Niacin (or Niaspan) is second best for lowering triglycerides if fibrates are not well tolerated.
- If you have a combination of high LDL and low HDL, Advicor (a combination of lovastatin and Niaspan) is the preferred choice in most cases.
- If you have a combination of high LDL and high Lp(a), Advicor is the preferred choice in most cases.
- If you have high LDL and small, dense LDL, Advicor or a statin paired with a fenofibrate is the preferred choice in most cases.

———— ◆•◆ ————

Chapter 12

Finding the Right Health Coach

Now that you have nearly completed this book, I hope you can appreciate the benefits of combining natural treatments with traditional care to optimize your heart disease prevention program. Your next step: finding a medical professional to help you put the pieces of your program together.

Of course, it's easy to find a cardiologist who follows the traditional approach to heart disease prevention—in other words, a doctor who will rely on standard cholesterol testing and treatment with prescription medication as the cornerstones of care. As you know from reading this book, however, traditional care very often does not go far enough. In order to minimize your risk, you need to identify and treat *all* your potential risk factors, including elevated CRP and Lp(a), undesirable LDL particle size, and other issues that a traditional doctor may not tell you about.

I believe that patients need a doctor with more than a prescription pad and a familiarity with cholesterol-lowering medications. I believe that every patient should have a health care "coach," someone who can help coordinate care from all helpful sources, whether traditional or alternative. The ideal health care team includes experts in nutrition, appropriate use of supplements, and mind–body techniques. These may include nutritionists, naturopaths, chiropractors, and acupuncturists, as well as practitioners of energy therapies, including healing touch and Reiki. Some medical doctors have experience and training in these disciplines, but far too many conventional doctors shun nontraditional healers. I have learned a great deal from experts in other health care arenas, and I believe my patients have benefited from my broader view of the healing process.

Far too often, patients who explore alternative health care options do so with little, if any, direction from their physicians. Worse yet, many patients never discuss these treatments with their doctors out of concern that the doctor will ridicule or abandon them if they reveal their involvement with alternative practitioners. I regret to say that these patients are right: Many doctors do condescend to patients who talk about alternative treatments, and some actually ask those patients to stop using complementary care or leave their practice. It is essential that you find a doctor with whom you share mutual trust and respect, and that includes someone who shares your overall philosophy of healing.

WHAT A GOOD DOCTOR LOOKS LIKE

Frankly, it's not always easy to find an open-minded physician. I suggest you settle for nothing less than one of the following:

- **The balanced healer.** This doctor is knowledgeable and has experience with a wide range of alternative and conventional approaches, and seeks to integrate the best of both worlds to achieve optimal results. He or she has obtained specialized training in alternative approaches, either in a formal program or via self-instruction. Unfortunately, there are currently very few formal training programs for physicians in this new combined approach, referred to as integrative medicine. The largest such program is at the University of Arizona and is directed by the highly respected Dr. Andrew Weil. You can find a listing of graduates from this program at http://integrativemedicine.arizona.edu/alum/index.html.

- **The open-minded physician.** This physician is not particularly knowledgeable about alternative approaches, but he or she is open to learning more and to working with you to explore natural options. This physician will make sure that you are not avoiding clearly indicated conventional therapies, will evaluate the available science surrounding selected alternative approaches, and will monitor your progress.

Consider how these two types of doctors might deal with a patient with high cholesterol who wanted to explore nonprescription options before resigning himself to lifelong use of statins. The balanced healer might have a detailed discussion with the patient about diet, including a comprehensive explanation of healthy and unhealthy fats. She might recommend a program that includes plant sterols and red yeast rice, or, alternatively, a low dose of a prescription statin in addition to coenzyme Q10. In addition, she might note that the patient experienced a lot of stress at home, which could be an additional cardiac risk factor; thus she might recommend biofeedback for stress reduction.

If that same patient visited an open-minded physician and

mentioned an article he read about the cholesterol-lowering properties of plant sterols, he might have a different experience. The open-minded physician might not be familiar with using plant sterols for cholesterol-reduction purposes, but he might do a quick medical literature review and learn that there is some evidence to support this approach. The open-minded physician might agree to watch the patient for three months or so while he takes plant sterols at the dosage supported by the literature. Upon retesting the patient's cholesterol levels, if the doctor finds that these levels have not declined to the desired goal, he might advise trying a more potent therapy.

Both of these doctors successfully manage the patient's cholesterol problem, and both respect the patient's eagerness to explore alternative therapies. In both scenarios, the patient receives excellent care and reduces his dependence on prescription medications. The patient's wishes and the doctor's expertise are respected, and, most importantly, the patient's cholesterol is brought into the target range.

AN OUNCE OF PREVENTION

When selecting a doctor, there's one other critical factor to consider: the doctor's emphasis on disease prevention. I often remind my patients that it's much easier to prevent heart disease than to deal with the consequences of a heart attack.

Regrettably, most doctors fail to emphasize the importance of prevention when talking to their patients. Heart disease prevention is quite complex, and new information is constantly emerging about both traditional and alternative care. As a result, preventive cardiology has become a specialty of its own.

If you have reason to be concerned about your risk of heart disease, I recommend that you choose a physician with a specialized focus on heart disease prevention. You may be able to get some idea about this based on discussions with friends or relatives, but you should be comfortable speaking to a prospective doctor directly about the issue. Don't be afraid to ask:

- Is a large part of your practice devoted solely to prevention?
- Do you order specialized blood tests when needed for risk factors that go beyond cholesterol? Do you test for CRP? Lp(a)? LDL particle size?
- Do you recommend the use of vitamins and nutritional supplements?
- If you believe I am a candidate for statin drugs but I do not tolerate or choose not to go on them, do you have experience with other treatment options?

In addition, when considering a doctor, you should also be sure to choose someone you feel comfortable working with. You should feel relaxed, listened to, and respected by your physician. If you do not, consider it a mismatch and keep looking. Despite the high-tech aspects of medicine today, the personal chemistry between the patient and doctor forms the foundation of a sound healing relationship.

Remember, you are the team captain, and your physician and other health care providers are all members of your team. If they are not helping you reach your goals, they need to play for another team. It's up to you to find the doctor who supports your health care vision, and one who shares your philosophical support of integrative medicine. The sense of empowerment you will feel at taking charge of your health care decisions will, in itself, be heart-healthy.

BE WELL

If you take care of your overall health, you're taking care of your heart as well. The evidence backs me up on this point: An analysis of the Nurses' Health Study estimated that fully 82 percent of cardiovascular events covered by the study could have been prevented by moderate diet and simple lifestyle modifications. In other words, cardiovascular disease is not an inevitable part of growing older.

I find this analysis incredibly uplifting: We have the power to make a huge difference in our health with the lifestyle choices we make. In my practice, I spotlight this sense of internal power by reminding my patients that they are their most important doctor, and that they are a more powerful healer than I—or any other physician—can be; all they need to do is fully realize their own healing abilities.

By taking the information in this book to heart and working with a physician who believes in an integrative approach to prevention, you can significantly improve your odds of avoiding a heart attack. I wish you nothing but happiness and good health in your journey.

Useful Internet Sites

———◆◆◆———

The following Web sites can be useful in learning about your cardiovascular health and general prevention strategies:

- www.americanheart.org. The American Heart Association Web site offers information on cholesterol, heart attack, and stroke. It sponsors the Cholesterol Low Down program, an online program designed to help individuals control their cholesterol.
- www.cdc.gov/nccdphp. The Centers for Disease Control and Prevention's National Center for Chronic Disease Prevention and Health Promotion offers a discussion on cardiovascular health. This site provides good background information, as well as national data on heart disease.
- www.drweil.com. This site offers valuable information about a wide range of prevention strategies, including nutrition, supplements, and mind–body approaches, from the leader of integrative medicine, Dr. Andrew Weil.
- http:nccam.nih.gov/health. The National Center for Complementary and Alternative Medicine's Web site

includes information about major areas of complementary and alternative medicine, including tips for finding practitioners, a medical journal search engine, and late-breaking medical news.

• www.nlm.nih.gov/medlineplus/coronarydisease.html. This highly recommended site contains selected heart-health topics from the National Library of Medicine at the National Institutes of Health. Focus sections include the latest news, diagnosis and symptoms, and prevention. In addition, the main National Library of Medicine site includes health-related new articles that are updated daily, as well as the PubMed research tool that allows visitors to search the archives of biomedical journal articles worldwide.

Chapter Notes

CHAPTER 2: Inflammation, Cholesterol, and Heart Disease

Berenson, G. S., et al. "Association Between Multiple Cardiovascular Risk Factors and Atherosclerosis in Children and Young Adults: The Bogalusa Heart Study." *New England Journal of Medicine,* 1998 June 4; 338 (23): 1650–6.

Joseph, A., Ackerman, D., et al. "Manifestations of Coronary Atherosclerosis in Young Trauma Victims: An Autopsy Study." *Journal of the American College of Cardiology,* 1993 August; 22 (2): 459–67.

Koro, C. E., et al. "The Independent Correlation Between High-Density Lipoprotein Cholesterol and Subsequent Major Adverse Coronary Events." *American Heart Journal,* 2006 March; 151 (3): 755,el–755e6.

Sharrett, A. R., et al. "Coronary Heart Disease Prediction From Lipoprotein Cholesterol Levels, Triglycerides, Lipoprotein(a), Apolipoproteins A-I and B, and HDL Density Subfractions: The Atherosclerosis Risk in Communities (ARIC) Study." *Circulation,* 2001 September 4; 104 (10): 1108–13.

Slapikas, R., et al. "Prevalence of Cardiovascular Risk Factors in

Coronary Heart Disease Patients with Different Low-Density Lipoprotein Phenotypes." *Medicina,* 2005; 41 (11): 925–31.

CHAPTER 3: Traditional Cholesterol Tests

Grundy, S., Cleeman, J., et al. "Implications of Recent Clinical Trials for the National Cholesterol Education Program Adult Treatment Panel III Guidelines." *Circulation,* 2004; 110: 227–39.

Heart Protection Study Collaborative Group. "MRC/BHF Heart Protection Study of Cholesterol Lowering with Simvastatin in 20,536 High-Risk Individuals: A Randomised Placebo-Controlled Trial." *Lancet,* 2002 July 6; 360 (9326): 7–22.

Ockene, I. S., et al. "Seasonal Variation in Serum Cholesterol Levels: Treatment Implications and Possible Mechanisms." *Archives of Internal Medicine,* 2004 April 26; 164 (8): 863–70.

Third Report of the National Cholesterol Education Program (NCEP) Expert Panel on Detection, Evaluation, and Treatment of High Blood Cholesterol in Adults (Adult Treatment Panel III), Executive Summary. Available at: www.nhlbi.nih.gov/guidelines/cholesterol/atp3xsum.pd.

Wiviott, S. D., et al. "Can Low-Density Lipoprotein Be Too Low? The Safety and Efficacy of Achieving Very Low Low-Density Lipoprotein with Intensive Statin Therapy: A PROVE IT-TIMI 22 Substudy." *Journal of the American College of Cardiology,* 2005 October 18; 46 (8): 1411–6.

CHAPTER 4: Digging Deeper

Albert, C. M., et al. "Prospective Study of C-Reactive Protein, Homocysteine, and Plasma Lipid Levels as Predictors of Sudden Cardiac Death." *Circulation,* 2002 June 4; 105 (22): 2595–9.

Albert, M. A., et al. "The Effect of Statin Therapy on Lipoprotein Associated Phospholipase A2 Levels." *Atherosclerosis,* 2005 September; 182 (1): 193–8.

Ariyo, A. A., et al. "Lp(a) Lipoprotein, Vascular Disease, and Mortality in the Elderly," *New England Journal of Medicine,* 2003 November 27; 349 (22): 2108–15.

Ballantyne, C. M., et al. "Lipoprotein-Associated Phospholipase A2, High-Sensitivity C-Reactive Protein, and Risk for Incident Coronary Heart Disease in Middle-Aged Men and Women in the Atherosclerosis Risk in Communities (ARIC) Study." *Circulation,* 2004 February 24; 109 (7): 837–42.

Bona, K. H., et al. "Homocysteine Lowering and Cardiovascular Events After Acute Myocardial Infarction." *New England Journal of Medicine,* 2006 March; 12: 354.

Dangas, G., et al. "Lipoprotein (a) and Inflammation in Human Coronary Atheroma." *Journal of the American College of Cardiology,* 1998 December; 32 (7): 2035–42.

Freedman, D. S., et al. "Sex and Age Differences in Lipoprotein Subclasses Measured by Nuclear Magnetic Resonance Spectroscopy: The Framingham Study." *Clinical Chemistry,* 2004 July; 50 (7): 1189–200.

Heart Outcome Prevention Evaluation (HOPE) Investigators. "Homocysteine Lowering with Folic Acid and B Vitamins in Vascular Disease." *New England Journal of Medicine,* 2006 March 12; 354.

Koenig, W., et al. "Lipoprotein-Associated Phospholipase A2 Plasma Concentrations Predict Cardiovascular Events in Patients with Coronary Heart Disease." *Journal of the American College of Cardiology,* 2005; 45 (Suppl A): A371.

Liu, S., et al. "Relation Between a Diet with a High Glycemic Load and Plasma Concentrations of High-Sensitivity C-Reactive Protein in Middle-Aged Women." *American Journal of Clinical Nutrition,* 2002; 75: 492–8.

Lopez-Garcia, E., et al. "Consumption of Trans Fatty Acids and

Plasma Markers of Inflammation and Endothelial Dysfunction." *Journal of Nutrition,* 2005; 135: 562–6.

Lue, G., et al. "Lipoprotein (a) as a Predictor of Coronary Heart Disease: The PRIME Study." *Atherosclerosis,* 2002 August; 163 (2): 377–84.

McCully, K. S. "Vascular Pathology of Homocysteinemia: Implications for the Pathogenesis of Arteriosclerosis." *American Journal of Pathology,* 1969; 26: 563–8.

Miller, D. T., et al. "Association of Common CRP Gene Variants with CRP Levels and Cardiovascular Events." *Annals of Human Genetics,* 2005 November; 69 (Pt 6): 623–38.

Nishina, P. M., et al. "Linkage of Atherogenic Lipoprotein Phenotype to the Low Density Lipoprotein Receptor Locus on the Short Arm of Chromosome 19." *Proceedings of the National Academy of Sciences, USA,* 1992 January 15; 89 (2): 708–12.

Rasouli, M. L., et al. "Plasma Homocysteine Predicts Progression of Atherosclerosis." *Atherosclerosis,* 2005 July; 181 (1): 159–65.

Ridker, P. M., et al. "Comparison of C-Reactive Protein and Low-Density Lipoprotein Cholesterol Levels in the Prediction of First Cardiovascular Events." *New England Journal of Medicine,* 2002 November 14; 347 (20): 1557–65.

Ridker, P. M., et al. "Inflammation, Aspirin, and the Risk of Cardiovascular Disease in Apparently Healthy Men." *New England Journal of Medicine,* 1997 April 3; 336 (14): 973–9.

Rifai, N. "Apolipoprotein (a) Size and Lipoprotein (a) Concentration and Future Risk of Angina Pectoria with Evidence of Severe Coronary Atherosclerosis in Men: The Physicians' Health Study." *Clinical Chemistry,* 2004 August; 50 (8): 1364–71.

Scanu, A. M. "Lipoprotein (a): A Genetic Risk Factor for Premature Coronary Heart Disease." *Journal of the American Medical Association,* 1992 June 24; 267 (24): 3326–9.

Sesso, H. H., et al. "C-Reactive Protein and the Risk of Developing Hypertension." *Journal of the American Medical Association,* 2003 December 10; 290 (22): 2945–51.

Shadid, S., et al. "Treatment of Obesity with Diet/Exercise Versus Pioglitazone Has Distinct Effects on Lipoprotein Particle Size." *Atherosclerosis,* 2005 November 25.

Stampfer, M. J., et al. "A Prospective Study of Plasma Homocysteine and Risk of Myocardial Infarction in US Physicians." *Journal of the American Medical Association,* 1992; 268: 877–81.

Stoney, C. M. "Plasma Homocysteine Levels Increase in Women During Psychological Stress." *Life Science,* 1999; 64 (25): 2359–65.

Superko, H. R. "The Atherogenic Lipoprotein Profile." *Science & Medicine,* 1998; 36–45.

Taylor, L. M., et al. "Prospective Blinded Study of the Relationship Between Plasma Homocysteine and Progression of Symptomatic Peripheral Arterial Disease." *Journal of Vascular Surgery,* 1999 January; 29 (1): 8–19.

Weil, Andrew. *Healthy Aging.* New York: Random House, 2005.

Williams, P. T., et al. "Smallest LDL Particles Are Most Strongly Related to Coronary Disease Progression in Men." *Arteriosclerosis, Thrombosis, and Vascular Biology,* 2003 February 1; 23 (2): 314–21.

Wood, R. J., et al. "Effects of a Carbohydrate-Restricted Diet on Emerging Plasma Markers for Cardiovascular Disease." *Nutrition and Metabolism* (London), 2006 May 4; 3 (1): 19.

CHAPTER 5: What You Can Learn from Heart Scans and Stress Tests

Greenland, P., et al. "Coronary Artery Calcium Score Combined with Framingham Score for Risk Prediction in Asymptomatic Individuals." *Journal of the American Medical Association,* 2004 February 4; 291 (2): 210–5.

Kondos, G. T., et al. "Electron-Beam Tomography Coronary

Artery Calcium and Cardiac Events." *Circulation,* 2003 May 27; 107: 25711–6.

Mahenthiran, J., et al. "Comparison of Prognostic Value of Stress Echocardiography Versus Stress Electrocardiography in Patients with Suspected Coronary Artery Disease." *American Journal of Cardiology,* 2005 September 1; 96 (5): 628–34.

Mollet, N. R., et al. "High-Resolution Spiral Computed Tomography Coronary Angiography in Patients Referred for Diagnostic Conventional Coronary Angiography." *Circulation,* 2005 October 11; 112 (15): 2318–23.

Sanfilippo, A. J., et al. "Stress Echocardiography in the Evaluation of Women Presenting with Chest Pain Syndrome: A Randomized, Prospective Comparison with Electrocardiographic Stress Testing." *Canadian Journal of Cardiology,* 2005 April; 21 (5): 405–12.

CHAPTER 6: Supplements for a Healthy Heart

Bona, K. H., et al. "Homocysteine Lowering and Cardiovascular Events After Acute Myocardial Infarction." *New England Journal of Medicine,* 2006 March 12; 354.

Burr, M. L. "Effects of Changes in Fat, Fish, and Fibre Intakes on Death and Myocardial Reinfarction: Diet and Reinfarction Trial (DART)." *Lancet,* 1989 September 30; 2 (8666): 757–61.

Dalen, J. E. "Aspirin to Prevent Heart Attack and Stroke: What's the Right Dose?" *American Journal of Medicine,* 2006 March; 119 (3): 198–202.

Guyton, J. R., et al. "Effectiveness of Once-Nightly Dosing of Extended-Release Niacin Alone and in Combination for Hypercholesterolemia." *American Journal of Cardiology,* 1998 September 15; 82 (6): 737–43.

Guyton, J. R., et al. "Extended-Release Niacin vs. Gemfibrozil for the Treatment of Low Levels of High-Density Lipoprotein Cholesterol." *Archives of Internal Medicine,* 2000 April 24; 160 (8): 1177–84.

Heart Outcome Prevention Evaluation (HOPE) Investigators. "Homocysteine Lowering with Folic Acid and B Vitamins in Vascular Disease." *New England Journal of Medicine,* 2006 March 12; 354.

Heber, D., et al. "Cholesterol-Lowering Effects of a Proprietary Chinese Red-Yeast-Rice Dietary Supplement." *American Journal of Clinical Nutrition,* 1999 February; 69 (2): 231–6.

Langsjoen, P., et al. "Treatment of Essential Hypertension with Coenzyme Q10." *Molecular Aspects of Medicine,* 1994; 15 Suppl: S265–72.

Lemaitre, R. N., et al. "n-3 Polyunsaturated Fatty Acids, Fatal Ischemic Heart Disease, and Nonfatal Myocardial Infarction in Older Adults: The Cardiovascular Health Study." *American Journal of Clinical Nutrition,* 2003 February; 77 (2): 319–25.

Loscalzo, Joseph. "Homocysteine Trials: Clear Outcomes for Complex Reasons." *New England Journal of Medicine,* 2006 March 12; 354.

Marckmann, P., et al. "Dietary Fish Oil (4 g Daily) and Cardiovascular Risk Markers in Healthy Men." *Arteriosclerosis, Thrombosis, and Vascular Biology,* 1997 December; 17 (12): 3384–91.

Miettinen, T. A., et al. "Reduction of Serum Cholesterol with Sitostanol-Ester Margarine in a Mildly Hypercholesterolemic Population." *New England Journal of Medicine,* 1995 November 16; 333 (20): 1350–1.

Morisco, C. "Effect of Coenzyme Q10 Therapy in Patients with Congestive Heart Failure: A Long-Term Multicenter Randomized Study." *Clinical Investigator,* 1993; 71 (8 Suppl): S134–6.

Neil, H. A., et al. "Randomised Controlled Trial of Use by Hypercholesterolaemic Patients of a Vegetable Oil Sterol-Enriched Fat Spread." *Atherosclerosis,* 2001 June; 156 (2): 329–37.

Pfeifer, M., et al. "Effects of a Short-Term Vitamin D_3 and Calcium Supplementation on Blood Pressure and Parathyroid Hormone Levels in Elderly Women." *Journal of Clinical Endocrinology and Metabolism,* 2001 April; 86 (4): 1633–7.

Scragg, R., et al. "Myocardial Infarction Is Inversely Associated with Plasma 25-Hydroxyvitamin D_3 Levels: A Community-Based Study." *International Journal of Epidemiology,* 1990 September; 19 (3): 559–63.

Singh, R. B., et al. "Effect of Coenzyme Q10 on Risk of Atherosclerosis in Patients with Recent Myocardial Infarction." *Molecular and Cellular Biochemistry,* 2003 April; 246 (1–2): 75–82.

Sirtori, C. R., et al. "L-Carnitine Reduces Plasma Lipoprotein (a) Levels in Patients with Hyper Lp (a)." *Nutrition, Metabolism, and Cardiovascular Disease,* 2000 October; 10 (5): 247–51.

CHAPTER 7: Eat Right

Albert, C. M., et al. "Nut Consumption and Decreased Risk of Sudden Cardiac Death in the Physicians' Health Study." *Archives of Internal Medicine,* 2002; 162: 1382–7.

Ascherio, A., et al. "Trans Fatty Acids and Coronary Heart Disease." *New England Journal of Medicine,* 1999; 340: 1994–8.

Bray, G. A., et al. "Consumption of High-Fructose Corn Syrup in Beverages May Play a Role in the Epidemic of Obesity." *American Journal of Nutrition,* 2004; (79): 537–43.

Elliott, S., et al. "Fructose, Weight Gain, and the Insulin Resistance Syndrome." *American Journal of Clinical Nutrition,* 2002; 76: 911–22.

Ganji, V., Kafai, M. R. "Frequent Consumption of Milk, Yogurt, Cold Breakfast Cereals, Peppers, and Cruciferous Vegetables and Intakes of Dietary Folate and Riboflavin but not Vitamins B_{12} and B_6 Are Inversely Associated with Serum Total Homocysteine Concentrations in the US Population." *American Journal of Clinical Nutrition,* 2004 December; 80 (6): 1500–7.

Hu, F., et al. "Dietary Fat Intake and the Risk of Coronary Heart Disease in Women." *New England Journal of Medicine,* 1997; 337: 1491–9.

Hu, F., et al. "Fish and Omega-3 Fatty Acid and Risk of Coronary Heart Disease in Women." *Journal of the American Medical Association,* 2002; 287: 1815–21.

Hu, F., et al. "Frequent Nut Consumption and Risk of Coronary Heart Disease: Prospective Cohort Study." *British Medical Journal,* 1998; 317: 1341–5.

Hu, F., Willett, W. "Optimal Diets for Prevention of Coronary Heart Disease." *Journal of the American Medical Association,* 2002 November 27; 288 (20): 2569–78.

Joshipura, K. J., et al. "The Effect of Fruit and Vegetable Intake on Risk for Coronary Heart Disease." *Annals of Internal Medicine,* 2001; 134: 1106–14.

Katan, M. B., Zock, P. L. "Trans Fatty Acids and Their Effects on Lipoproteins in Humans." *Annual Review of Nutrition,* 1995; 15: 473–93.

Liu, S., et al. "A Prospective Study of Dietary Fiber Intake and Risk of Cardiovascular Disease Among Women." *Journal of the American College of Cardiology,* 2002; 39: 49–56.

Liu, S., et al. "A Prospective Study of Dietary Glycemic Load and Risk of Myocardial Infarction in Women." *American Journal of Clinical Nutrition,* 2000; 71: 1455–61.

Liu, S., et al. "Relation Between a Diet with a High Glycemic Load and Plasma Concentrations of High-Sensitivity C-Reactive Protein in Middle-Aged Women." *American Journal of Clinical Nutrition,* 2002 March; 75 (3): 492–8.

Mensink, R. P., Katan, M. B. "Effect of Dietary Trans Fatty Acids on High-Density and Low-Density Lipoprotein Cholesterol Levels in Healthy Subjects." *New England Journal of Medicine,* 1990; 323: 439–45.

Mozaffarian, D., et al. "Dietary Intake of Trans Fatty Acids and Systemic Inflammation in Women." *American Journal of Clinical Nutrition,* 2004 April; 79: 606–12.

Stampfer, M. J., et al. "Primary Prevention of Coronary Heart Disease in Women Through Diet and Lifestyle." *New England Journal of Medicine,* 2000; 343: 16–22.

Summers, L. K., et al. "Substituting Dietary Saturated Fat with Polyunsaturated Fat Changes Abdominal Fat Distribution and Improves Insulin Sensitivity." *Diabetologia,* 2002; 45: 369–77.

Sundram, K., et al. "Trans (Elaidic) Fatty Acids Adversely Affect the Lipoprotein Profile Relative to Specific Saturated Fatty Acids in Humans." *Journal of Nutrition,* 1997; 127: 514S–20S.

Weil, Andrew. *Healthy Aging.* New York: Random House, 2005.

CHAPTER 8: Mind–Body Approaches to a Healthy Heart

Bijlani, R. L., et al. "A Brief but Comprehensive Lifestyle Education Program Based on Yoga Reduces Risk Factors for Cardiovascular Disease and Diabetes Mellitus." *Journal of Alternative and Complementary Medicine,* 2005 April; 11 (2): 267–74.

Das, S., O'Keefe, J. H. "Behavioral Cardiology: Recognizing and Addressing the Profound Impact of Psychosocial Stress on Cardiovascular Health." *Current Atherosclerosis Report,* 2006 March; 8 (2): 111–8.

Luskin, F. "Review of the Effect of Spiritual and Religious Factors on Mortality and Morbidity with a Focus on Cardiovascular and Pulmonary Disease." *Journal of Cardiopulmonary Rehabilitation,* 2000 January–February; 20 (1): 8–15.

Mamtani, R., et al. "Ayurveda and Yoga in Cardiovascular Diseases." *Cardiology in Review,* 2005 May–June; 13 (3): 155–62.

Steptoe, A., Brydon, L. "Associations Between Acute Lipid Stress Responses and Fasting Lipid Levels 3 Years Later." *Health Psychology,* 2005; 24 (6): 601–7.

Weil, Andrew. *Breathing: The Master Key to Self Healing* (audio book). Boulder, CO: Sounds True, Inc., 1999.

CHAPTER 9: Exercise

Brochu, M., et al. "Modest Effects of Exercise Training Alone on Coronary Risk Factors and Body Composition in Coronary Patients." *Journal of Cardiopulmonary Rehabilitation,* 2000 May–June; 20 (3): 180–8.

Chek, P. *How to Eat, Move, and Be Healthy!* A C.H.E.K. Institute Publication, 2004.

Tanasescu, M., et al. "Exercise Type and Intensity in Relation to Coronary Heart Disease in Men." *Journal of the American Medical Association,* 2002 October 23; 288 (16): 1994–2000.

Tokmakidis, S. P., Volaklis, K. A. "Training and Detraining Effects of a Combined-Strength and Aerobic Exercise Program on Blood Lipids in Patients with Coronary Artery Disease." *Journal of Cardiopulmonary Rehabilitation,* 2003 May–June; 23 (3): 193–200.

CHAPTER 10: Quitting Smoking

Blondal, T., et al. "Nicotine Nasal Spray with Nicotine Patch for Smoking Cessation: Randomised Trial with Six Year Follow Up." *British Journal of Medicine,* 1999 January 30; 318 (7179): 285–8.

Jorenby, D. E., et al. "A Controlled Trial of Sustained-Release Bupropion, a Nicotine Patch, or Both for Smoking Cessation." *New England Journal of Medicine,* 1999 March 4; 340 (9): 685–91.

Ockene, I., Miller, N. H. "Cigarette Smoking, Cardiovascular Disease, and Stroke: A Statement for the American Heart Association Task Force on Risk Reduction." *Circulation,* 1997; 96: 3243–7.

Spiegel, D., et al. "Predictors of Smoking Abstinence Following a Single-Session Restructuring Intervention with Self-Hypnosis." *American Journal of Psychiatry,* 1993; 150: 1090–7.

Stewart, J. H. "Hypnosis in Contemporary Medicine." *Mayo Clinic Proceedings,* 2005 April; 80 (4): 511–24.

Tekawa, I., Friedman, S. "Effect of Cigar Smoking on the Risk of Cardiovascular Disease, Chronic Obstructive Pulmonary Disease, and Cancer in Men." *New England Journal of Medicine,* 1999 June 10; 340 (23): 1773–80.

Viswesvaran, C., Schmidt, F. L. "A Meta-Analytic Comparison of the Effectiveness of Smoking Cessation Methods." *Journal of Applied Psychology,* 1992 August; 77 (4): 554–61.

CHAPTER 11: When to Consider Medication for Cholesterol Treatment

Albert, M. A., et al. "Effect of Statin Therapy on C-Reactive Protein Levels: The Pravastatin Inflammation CRP Evaluation (PRINCE)." *Journal of the American Medical Association,* 2001; 286: 64–70.

Jones, P. H., Davidson, M. H. "Reporting Rate of Rhabdomyolysis with Fenofibrate + Statin Versus Gemfibrozil + Any Statin." *American Journal of Cardiology,* 2005 January 1; 95 (1): 120–2.

Ray, K. K., et al. "Relationship Between Uncontrolled Risk Factors and C-Reactive Protein Levels in Patients Receiving Standard or Intensive Statin Therapy for Acute Coronary Syndromes in the PROVE IT–TIMI 22 Trial." *Journal of the American College of Cardiology,* 2005 October 18; 46 (8): 1417–24.

Ridker, P. M., et al. "C-Reactive Protein Levels and Outcomes After Statin Therapy." *New England Journal of Medicine,* 2005 January 6; 352(1): 20–8.

Stampfer, M. J. "Primary Prevention of Coronary Heart Disease in Women Through Diet and Lifestyle." *New England Journal of Medicine,* 2000 July 6; 343 (1): 16–22.

Yeh, E., Willerson, J. "Coming of Age of C-Reactive Protein: Using Inflammation Markers in Cardiology." *Circulation,* 2003 January 28; 107: 370–2.

Index

About the Author

STEPHEN DEVRIES, MD, is director of the Integrative Program for Heart Disease Prevention at the University of Illinois, Chicago, and medical director of the University of Illinois Healthy Heart Center in Deerfield, Illinois. He is also associate professor of clinical medicine at the University of Illinois, Chicago. Dr. Devries is a diplomate of the American Board of Internal Medicine, subspecialty cardiovascular disease, and a fellow of the American Society of Echocardiography. Dr. Devries authored the weekly column "Heart Beat" in the *Chicago Sun-Times,* and lectures nationally on prevention of heart disease. He completed an associate fellowship in integrative medicine at the University of Arizona under the direction of Dr. Andrew Weil. Dr. Devries was voted by his peers to be one of "the Best Doctors in America, 2005–2006." He can be contacted through his Web site, www.healthyheartcenter.com.